The Pastoral Role in Caring for the Dying and Bereaved

The Foundation of Thanatology Series, Volume 7

Other Volumes in the Series

The Pastoral Role in Caring for the Dying and Bereaved

Pragmatic and Ecumenical

edited by
Brian P. O'Connor
Daniel J. Cherico
Carole E. Smith Torres
Austin H. Kutscher
Jacob Goldberg
Karin M. Muraszko

with the assistance of
Lillian G. Kutscher

PRAEGER

New York
Westport, Connecticut
London

BV
4335
.P377
1986

Library of Congress Cataloging-in-Publication Data

The Pastoral role in caring for the dying and
bereaved.

(The Foundation of Thanatology series ; v.7)

Includes index.
1. Pastoral medicine—Addresses, essays, lectures.
2. Church work with the terminally ill—Addresses,
essays, lectures. 3. Church work with the bereaved—
Addresses, essays, lectures. 4. Death—Religious
aspects—Christianity—Addresses, essays, lectures.
5. Bereavement—Religious aspects—Christianity—
Addresses, essays, lectures. I. O'Connor, Brian,
1945-   . II. Kutscher, Lillian G. III. Series:
Foundation of Thanatology series (Praeger Publishers);
v.3.
BV4335.P377   1986   253.5   86-545
ISBN 0-275-92153-0   (alk. paper)

Library of Congress Catalog Card Number: 86-545
ISBN: 0-275-92153-0

First published in 1986

Praeger Publishers, 521 Fifth Avenue, New York, NY 10175
A division of Greenwood Press, Inc.

Printed in the United States of America

The paper used in this book complies with the
Permanent Paper Standard issued by the National
Information Standards Organization (Z39.48-1984).

10 9 8 7 6 5 4 3 2 1

Thanatology is a discipline whose focus is on the practice of supportive physical and emotional care for those who are life-threatened, with an equal concern exhibited for the well-being of their family members. Proposed is a philosophy of care-giving that reinforces alternative ways of enhancing the quality of life, that introduces methods of intervention on behalf of the emotional status of all involved, that fosters a more mature understanding of the dying process and the problems of separation, loss, bereavement, and grief.

The editors wish to acknowledge the support and encouragement of the Foundation of Thanatology in the preparation of this book. All royalties from its sale are directly assigned to this not-for-profit, tax-exempt, public, scientific, and educational foundation.

Contents

Introduction

Brian P. O'Connor

A number of years ago, I spoke to a family regarding a sick relative. I mentioned to them that the physicians were advising further consultations with a specialist. Almost in unison, the family groaned: "Not another specialist . . . God deliver us from specialists." Somehow, the word "specialist" had a pejorative connotation for this family.

In the last few years, we have seen much in the health literature that speaks about holistic medicine. The whole patient and the family has become the unit of care in our health facilities, not just that "part" of the person under the care of a specialist. I believe that it is this trend that prompts people to reject the notion of "cure" in favor of the all-encompassing idea of "care." If there is any word that adequately describes this concept of care or concern for the whole person, it is the term "pastoral." I have not heard anyone accuse a member of a pastoral team of being a "specialist." However, that does not mean that the pastoral care-giver is unprofessional or unqualified.

What does it mean to be a "pastoral" care-giver? Can such a person be described as a visitor to the sick, a hand-holder, or a well-intentioned paraprofessional? I believe that the key element in pastoral care is a person's ability to free others from the obstacles or restrictions that prevent them from appreciating the reality that they truly are sons and daughters of a loving, forgiving God. What better specialty can one hope to practice?

All of us may at times question the effectiveness of what we do as professionals. The teacher begins to feel that real education is something in the past, the physician may feel that medicine is ultimately fighting a losing battle, the author may feel that words are wasted on a visual society. The affirmations that encourage teacher, physician, and author to continue with their trades are often contained within society itself. The student who excels, the patient who walks, the reader who laughs--these are antidotes for apathy and indifference for the professional. Unfortunately, many in our society do not bother to see the successes of pastoral care. Religion is nice for many but it is not on the same level with oncology, nuclear medicine, and so forth, when it comes to helping people. Often, the pastoral success stories make for good case histories but lack the professional aspect of care. This book is an attempt to furnish all of us with the tools of pastoral care and the insight that comes from actually seeing the successes of our profession.

When we use the word "pragmatic," we do not want to speak as if it is the opposite of "professional." Rather, the pragmatic approach of pastoral care grounds us very concretely to "hands-on" care. So many of the concepts we have regained in health care relate directly to the pastoral approach. I vividly remember the stage routine of Father Malcolm Boyd a few years ago. He spoke about his own approach to patients in a hospital setting--the power of touch--not to examine but to join; the power of care--to listen; the power of doing simple things--unwrapping the fruit, cleaning the waste basket, giving water. This approach to care struck me as the way God comes to us in a pastoral way. In thinking about care for others, I also recall the description of Bishop Fulton J. Sheen when he spoke about his heart operation. He mentioned waking up in the cardiac care unit of Lenox Hill Hospital in New York City and seeing a figure walking between the beds. He suddenly felt very happy because he envisioned this figure as being that of God passing through all the intensive care units of the world and telling the sick to place their pains and sufferings on his shoulders so that he might carry them. Sheen acknowledged that he was a much better minister to the sick after this experience; he knew that his role was to aid and assist a God who worked at caring, loving, and forgiving.

Good pastoral care demands that we fully develop our gifts to counsel and soothe the broken-hearted. The tools of psychiatry and other similar disciplines can only make us better practitioners of our art. However, the aim of pastoral care must never be forgotten. We are helping to free ourselves and others of the demons inside of us in order to appreciate the presence of God. The liberation from difficulties is not an end in itself but the setting of the stage for a greater understanding of God's presence within us. The tools of psychiatry empower us to reveal more clearly the face of the God of Abraham, Isaac, and Jacob.

How important is the task of a pastoral minister to the sick and the dying? How vital is this function in the whole fabric of human existence? In answering these questions, let me borrow from a description often quoted by Rabbi Jacob Goldberg. In Psalm 147, 1-4, we read: "Praise the Lord, for he is good; sing praise to our God, for he is gracious, it is fitting to praise him. The Lord rebuilds Jerusalem; the dispersed of Israel he gathers. He heals the broken-hearted and binds up their wounds. He tells the number of the stars, he calls each by name." God brings back the exiles to a rebuilt Jerusalem and creates the universe. Liberation and creation: obviously two important works of God. Between these two works, we see listed another: healing and binding the wounded. Does pastoral care of the sick and the dying need any better justification than what is spelled out in God's word? Our God creates, saves, and heals our wounds.

Part I

An Overview of the Pastoral Role

1

Clergy and the Consumer

Carole E. Smith Torres

One of the most significant issues facing today's professional minister is understanding the nature and purpose of the religious community in society. The religious community is unable to function according to biblical and traditional design because of outside pressures that force it to reflect an institutional structure. Many advocate a spiritual leadership based on sophisticated management theories and techniques; the Scriptures beckon us to rediscover the religious community's structure and function as planned and executed by God.

What is the ultimate function of the clergy? How can our lives reflect the love, caring, discipline, and guidance that we find in Scripture? Are these not the ultimate strengths of our being made in the image of God? The concept of religious community as a sharing, caring people, not as an institution, provides the framework within which our response to those with life-threatening or acute illnesses can be made.

We write and speak of what we can do. We need to ex-press in a more tangible way that we are a people who care for the hurting lovingly and supportively.

A universal set of reactions results from the threats inherent in acute illness. Consequently, a variety of important needs arise--not only for the ill but for the family members as well. But changes in the pattern of life within our culture over the past few decades have tended to multiply the frequency and severity of these needs.

Kübler-Ross (1975) has described the hospitalization experiences of dying patients as depersonalizing within an environment that does not meet the entire spectrum of those human needs arising from disease. In fact, the terminal or chronically ill patient often represents "failure" to many in the medical profession. Although technologically equipped for healing, doctors are unable to help their patients with more

3

"sublime" needs--that is, giving life, and giving life meaning.
The doctor is not God!

PATIENT FEELINGS

A person living with physical or emotional trauma feels
isolated. The resultant impact on the individual is destructive.
Institutional systems and procedures effectively deny the individual a personal sense of identity, control, or status. Feelings of embarrassment, inferiority, and the focus of attention
on the patient's body have a debilitating effect on the patient's self-esteem. As the object of tests and examinations
and sterile routines, the person consequently withdraws into
a variety of self-protective behaviors. There is also a sense
of oppression, fear, and anxiety that can easily be followed
by depression. All of this, coupled with the actual pain of
illness and the threat of death can initiate self-pity as a new
way of life.

Many helpers find latent fears about illness and death
stirred within them. Who wants to face the reality of one's
own death? Most people do not know what to say to those who
are dying, or how to relate to them--this includes clergy!
The clergy are also pressed with the normal pressures of
scheduling, not enough time to visit, as well as the deep desire not to get involved. And how many times are human beings emotionally mature enough themselves to walk through
the experience of suffering with someone who is thus afflicted?

Religion has always been concerned with helping people
develop major insights and perspectives on life. Dr. Edgar
Jackson has lectured that

> whatever the religion, it is in essence designed
> to help people cope with all of life's experiences.
> . . .One of the things that is basic to any re-
> ligious perspective is theology . . . a religious
> philosophy, a way of looking at life so that one
> can deal with all there is of life.

My own world view and religious philosophy or theology
derives from an investigation of the Scriptures--both the Old
and New Testaments. As I have exegeted the text--closely
examined it and tried to apply it to our own age and to my
own life specifically--I have found basic and vital truths communicated. These have been foundational to my working with
others. This ancient, timeless text, the Bible, asserts that
God has created both the universe and us, has set His love
and affection on us, has overseen history, and has deep purposes for each human being. On the sacred page, one learns
that man has dignity because he is created in the image of
God.

These truths are not only foundational to my work; they form the basis of a concrete answer to the many painful questions that come with life--questions that I have pondered; mysteries I have grappled with, and still find myself wrestling with. To those with whom I work, I wish to present God as a source of hope, life, and peace, even though they may be suffering. I emphasize that He is not socially removed from the scene of pain and grief. Rather, God is touched with the feeling of our infirmities. He has historically identified himself with the plight of mankind.

Cultural changes have their impact. Today's "family" is, in most cases, a nuclear unit. While the extended family may in fact be closely tied emotionally, the small immediate family is still isolated. When physical disability interrupts the family's lifestyle, too heavy an emotional load is placed on this small unit. Yet family members must be acquainted with the psychological pressures facing the patient and play significant supportive roles. In the past, the function of religion was to provide help for people coping with life's deepest problem.

THE CLERGY'S TASK

The clergy must strive to develop sensitivity and minister to people as whole persons. There is a great need for more sensitive care by clergy who understand the special concern of those who are suffering. Some skills to develop include: (1) an appropriately caring attitude, sympathy coupled with empathy; (2) an ability to communicate God's love effectively and realistically in a practical way; (3) an ability to share a dimension of hope, so essential to help the patient "keep on going;" and (4) the ability to restrain from giving easy answers.

In all ages, attempts have been made to define who man is. The most complete picture, I believe, is given in the Scriptures: man is noble, yet fallen; creative and sufficient in many ways. Yet man requires God as a vital necessity in order to be loved unconditionally, to have meaning and purpose, to know freedom from guilt (forgiveness), and to know freedom from anxiety. The Scriptures speak to every human need and problem: loneliness, grief, betrayal, loss, and physical and emotional pain. With this comes the astounding, almost too good to be true promise that through an all-powerful, all-knowing, compassionate God these needs can be met unequivocally.

The New Testament gives the added dimension that forgiveness and life come through the person of Jesus Christ. Here we read that death need no longer have the same sting --the fear of death has been dealt with through Jesus Christ, who conquered death through the resurrection. Other suggestions include the ability to offer support, faith, and fact; to deal with fears and futility; to give future hope. There is stability derived from assurance that He will fulfill, a belief based upon theological and historical fact.

Clergy represent God to others, and this is an awesome responsibility. They must be prepared to deal with various types of emotional expressions, including the patient's anger, not only against the clergy but also ultimately against God. Reflection on the positive side of suffering is not inappropriate. The critically ill person has a great deal of time to think about the deeper things of life: Why was I created? Is there a God? How can I change my priorities? Can I change my priorities now that time is short? Can I still be able to give in a significant way? I want to know I have something to give as one who is going through suffering.

The clergy can encourage the hidden potential within a sick person. They can encourage laughter and humor in appropriate ways to comfort the person. When those who are suffering see life through a dark tunnel, the clergy must help them to see the light that is at the end of that tunnel. If our God is impotent in our own minds and hearts, we as God's representatives will be impotent proportionately.

We must acknowledge the importance of genuineness and warmth in the caring relationship. Will ill persons want this kind of relationship? Will they want to talk about their illness or their future? Will they reject our overtures of comfort? Will they make matters worse? What can we say that will truly help and encourage?

Our unfamiliarity with illness and death--by their nature they isolate the patient from the normal pattern of life-- deepens our uncertainty and increases our hesitation in becoming involved with those held in the clutch of severe illness. If clergy are to grow as helping persons, and if our congregations are to grow as caring communities, we must face such fears about suffering. Only in this way can we affirm the value of each person and help make passage through the valley a part of growth toward God as well as achievement of full potential as a person.

2

The Identity and Role of Clergy

Gordon E. Jackson

THE CLERGYPERSON'S IDENTITY

Identity is currently such a fashionable word, both within and outside of psychological circles, that some might avoid it if they could. But in order to define the role of the clergy, we need to ask about clergy identity, since that has come into serious question for individual members of the clergy, the religious community, and society in general.

Who are those who minister to dying patients and their families? They have formal status as the chaplains, pastors, or priests of some churches, or as the rabbis of synagogues. However, along with the general diminution of status in our society, clergy ecclesiastical status is becoming less impressive. Most clergy have limited professional training. Within the last 30 years, that training has usually included a course or two in the theory and practice of pastoral care, interlaced with some borrowings from the behavioral sciences, especially depth psychology. Some clergy have been seduced by the sirens of an appealing scientific empiricism; others, fearing some kind of compromise of faith, have sought safety in obscurantism; still others have steered what I regard as a correct course, using the findings of the behavioral sciences without losing sight of their theological direction. However, ecclesiastical status and professional training are precursors to identity, not identity itself.

When members of the clergy are with the dying and the grieving, they are expected to have insight into those values that are regarded as ultimate or at least supremely worthwhile, as well as insight into the spoilers of those values--guilt, estrangement, and death. The clergy are expected to provide caring that brings some curing to the

minds and hearts, if not the bodies of those who are dying
and grieving.

I am not satisfied with a representative definition of
identity nor with an identity defined by role expectations,
important as they are. No doubt clergy are marked by both
of these identities. What seems more significant is the internalized identity of individual clerics. Out of the billions
of events that have crowded them over the space of years,
including both the events they have rejected and those to
which they have conformed, and out of the host of possibilities that constantly beckon them, how have they put themselves together so that they are particular, unique persons?
What is the content of that uniqueness? What are the qualities that have endured through time that identify these individuals? In Whiteheadian terms, have they created out of the
vast multiplicity of their environments selves that are beautiful, that have brought and continue to bring harmony out of
contrasts, and developed depth instead of allowing trivia to
flatten their lives? In Jungian terms, have they individuated
out of a constant dialogue between the conscious and the unconscious poles? In Freudian terms, have they sorted out the
myriad introjects that form the memory traces of their minds?
Have they discriminated among the introjects to form a clear
hierarchy of values? Have they, to borrow from Sartre, made
some of those values the "projects" of their lives? As myth-
makers--and we all are--have they constructed their myths
so that they are windows on reality, even if reality beggars
precise description? And is their faith malleable enough to
cope with change and strong enough to cope with death, the
final form of change? However, these questions are really
rhetorical. Fundamentally, the identity of clerics is who they
have become by working through their own commitments and
their own belief systems about the ultimate meaning of life,
suffering, and death.

When they walk into hospital rooms or funeral homes
what they bring is themselves: visible, open, awesome selves
who are present to others. They have no medical instruments,
no trays laden with medications. They may carry no Bible
or prayer book although, if these objects correlate with their
individual being, they can speak that being powerfully. This
does not imply the personhood of others is not important. My
contention is that, to dying patients and their families, what
clerics have internalized and made their own is fundamentally
what they have to offer in the caring role. Allport's (1967)
distinction between intrinsic and extrinsic religionists is the
distinction being made here. Finally, religious crutches and
externalized support systems prove inferior. The identity of
the individual cleric is what the person intrinsically is; and
what the person intrinsically is, is for the dying and the
grieving.

Therefore, a crucial concern is what feeds the cleric's life. (This is, of course, crucial to the life of every person, but we are now addressing the clergy.) The background for caring in public moments is their private caring for their own souls, whether in private or in the intimate support groups that nourish them gently and honestly. Pastoral care begins with their care of themselves, which is too often jettisoned in a highly technological, frenzied society. Pastoral care in the midst of any serious loss, but especially death, requires faithful homework out of which an intrinsic quality of peace in the sense of wholeness can emerge.

CLERGY IDENTITY AND ROLE: PLURALISTIC BELIEF SYSTEMS

If the identity of clergy members is fundamentally an intrinsic identity, dependent on how each has woven the tapestry of individual being out of the myriad threads of relationships, how does the identity serve any pastoral caring situation with integrity, especially that circling death, given the pluralistic belief systems of our society? The pastoral role is obviously made more difficult by this pluralism. Within a context of pervasive secularity and confronted by a tremendous range of religious object-choices, members of the clergy have serious problems. Can they remain faithful to their own faith and yet respect with integrity the belief systems of others? If so, do they require a secular priesthood borrowed from other disciplines, such as social work or psychiatry? The major concern must be dying patients and their families, whose value systems must be respected within any pastoral caring.

It is my considered judgment that only by remaining faithful to our own religious commitments can we respect with integrity the belief systems of dying patients or their families. If we do not have respect for our own integrity, we will not have respect for theirs. It would be immoral to proselytize dying patients. Surely our language is not so stilted nor our symbols so parochial that we need different communicative signs for deeply human communication.

Since the clergy's role is essentially religious, we must ask what it is to be religious in the setting of death and dying. Minimally, it is that we humans are of primary value, that we have, in the words of Becker (1971), "cosmic specialness," that we have some meaning that outlasts time as we know it. It should be noted that I have attached no god or god-talk to this minimal understanding. Theological language is critical, because God is essential in the clergy's understanding of reality. But, for the moment, religious value has to do phenomenologically with what is primitively meaningful to the human person. How to affirm the religious primacy of

the narcissistic human self and to give that primacy an onto-
logical hope is the clergy's fundamental problem. I maintain
that all clergypersons who have reflected on the human scene
should be able to help almost any patient with this basic affirmation. Further, I believe that they will find in the incredible richness of human experience those symbols of hope that
can enhance dying patients' struggles for primary value and
their families' ambivalent struggles for their own continuing
self-affirmation and identity. I, who believe in God with many
of the traditional symbols excised, believe that because God
does not have problems about religion, as we do, God is not
disturbed by our inarticulateness or by the confusion among
our many symbolic systems. God is aching over the suffering
and dying of each of us as we struggle to affirm our onto-
logical value in the face of what would threaten to extinguish
that value. The clergy need to remember that God is not going to suffer a narcissistic wound because somehow we have
failed in our compulsion to name Him. His wound is the anguish of dying patients and their grieving families. Yet to
name God, to introduce that powerful name at the intuited
and appropriate moment, is to lift anguish and grief into a
presence that can breathe hope into the pathos of the existential pain.

That pain needs the comfort of hope, a hope that is
both penultimate and ultimate. Penultimate hopes are those
engendered by human community. The clergy are freed by a
congregation of people to spend time with the dying and the
grieving. They are also freed, ostensibly, from crippling denial, so that they are willing to spend time with the dying
and the grieving. As a dying man told his wife the morning
after a late-night vigil by his pastor: "He sat there--all
night. He didn't leave me." A bit of one life fed into the
dying man's life, bringing surcease from night terror and,
for a time, maybe even peace. Penultimate hopes sometimes
point to ultimate hope.

When Weisman (1972) said "hope is . . . the basic
assumption in living and dying . . ." he was in agreement
with theologians from most of the great world religions. It
seems to me that there is a trajectory in human life named
hope, which clergy can presuppose. When clergy affirm in
noncoercive ways that at the center of things there is a con-
serving love that saves everything savable out of this ambiguous life, we are on target with that inner trajectory toward
ultimate hope. Thus, one function of religion is to keep hope
open to a limitless future that defies our finitude by the full
transcendence of almost unimaginable possibility. The role of
clerics is to point to the "almost unimaginable," to be the
nourishers of hope. However, this role presupposes that they
have, to some significant degree, worked through the curriculum of their lives and gained individual identities that

help articulate and authenticate the support they bring, especially as they point toward the source of ultimate hope.

TWO PASTORAL ROLES FOR DEATH, DYING, AND GRIEVING

A Teaching Responsibility

Long before a crisis occurs, clergy have a pedagogical responsibility to help prepare people to face their own death and those of others. Whitehead (1979) reminds us in his process philosophy that all of life is a "perpetual perishing." Small losses should help us to get ready for larger ones, gradual separations for abrupt and final ones, some grief for much grief. The raw experience of a constant dying, from present moments slipping forever into the past to traumatic moments of physical death, is the ground from which meaning about life and death should grow and mature.

Churches and synagogues are the chief teaching institutions in which people might be helped to see that death is a part of life. This is not an exercise is morbidity but rather a teaching about mortality. We humans seem to spend so much of life serving an infantile wish for omnipotence. Clergy can best serve the pedagogical role when they stress human finitude and mortality through preaching, teaching, and general caring. The church and synagogue should be fairly safe contexts in which to provide reminders of mortality that are good, and of finitude that can afford to relax within an infinite love. Then illusion will have less of a future and denial a less powerful defense. Would it not be a magnificent contribution for the clergy to help us all give death the place in our thought and life that belongs to it? If we could all be helped to imagine our own death, to take that event up into ourselves as a component of the fullness of our lives, we would be helped toward the acceptance of our own death and the deaths of our loved ones.

Crisis Intervention

What, specifically, is the role of clergy members when they are involved in crisis intervention with dying patients and their families? First, it is caring that goes out to meet the other as a Thou. In Martin Buber's category of I-Thou, two subjects meet. Clerics do not treat patients impersonally, as medical teams usually do. The cleric meets the other in the reality that they now share, the reality of dying. The pastoral carer is there not to deny death, but to affirm the dying one. It is a dying patient's subjectivity that the clergy move out to meet. The clergy are professional enough to know what's going on and not to be afraid or timid about it; professional enough to know the techniques for reading the body's language, and to watch for hidden agendas; professional enough to know that the timing of questions or remarks is of the essence. But they do not allow professionalism to get in the way of the other role.

This is the critical role of the clergy. The hospital staff may be too busy or too denying, the family too engrossed in separation anxiety and denial, friends too apprehensive and too removed. Clergy members are there in the nakedness of their humanity to meet dying people in the nakedness of their humanity. It may be the simple question proposed by Kübler-Ross, "How sick are you?" that makes possible a first disclosure: "I am full of cancer!" In a real meeting between the clergyperson and the patient, the patient's fears, anxieties, and sense of alienation, as well as unasked questions and unspoken needs, will have a chance to emerge. If the clergyperson runs away from this I-Thou relationship, the patient is denied one more opening onto a poignant, possibly redemptive, real-life encounter. The tragedy is that there may be few such openings left.

I wince when I recall that last evening with my friend I was going out of town for a few days, but told him I would see him as soon as I returned. He said, "I may be moved before then." I heard the deeper word, but responded to the surface word. "Oh, I'll find you," I said. He was tired and closed his eyes. I knew I had missed him. The moment had passed. The art of pastoral caring is intervention that is not coercive but gentle and patient-centered, creating a genuine I-Thou meeting so that spirit can create peace along the concourse yet to be lived.

So often, however, clergy cannot help patients in a really meaningful way if they do not include their families. Studies on death and dying indicate that it is the family that often keeps dying patients from separating from their environment. The normal, healthy detachment of the dying is made more painful by family demands that "you have to get well," and by pretenses that "you're looking so much better." The family holds on when the patient may want and need to let go and die in peace. Clergy can often be constructive third parties who can interpret to families the psychospiritual needs of the dying. The pastor's listening, a moral obligation as well as an art, can help the work of grief to begin by eliciting the anger and tending the pain of separation. Some precious moments between patient and family can be a sublime reality through the clergy's facilitating role of bringing them together in a dialogue of feeling, gesture, and word. The clergyperson's work, if begun in the pathos of ebbing life and continued through the benumbing activities of the funeral, has the best chance of contributing to grief work through family care after the patient has died. The clergyperson has the unique opportunity to provide continuity of healing until reality has once more become secure.

Neither patients nor families expect of clergy the miracles they expect of medical doctors. They only expect evidence of a sensitive concern; therein is the hidden skill of the fine art of caring. The rituals of pastoral caring, validated over the centuries, must be constantly revalidated by the best theory we know and by sensitive reference to dying patients and grieving families. Prayer books and Scriptures can be not only the means to peace, but defense against our anxiety. The quality of caring offers patients and their families the possibility of those rare but redemptive moments when people meet and, in meeting, know themselves to be validated. Such validation is a ground of peace for those who are dying and for those who grieve.

REFERENCES

Allport, G. The Individual and His Religion. New York: Macmillan, 1967.

Becker, E. The Birth and Death of Meaning, 2nd ed. New York: Free Press, 1971.

Bolsen, A. Exploration of the Inner World: A Study of Mental Disorder and Religious Experience. Philadelphia: University of Pennsylvania Press, 1971.

--- and Leary, J. Religion in Crisis and Custom: A Sociological Study. Westport, Conn.: Greenwood Press, 1973.

Kübler-Ross, E. On Death and Dying. New York: Macmillan, 1969.

Weisman, A.D. On Dying and Denying. A Psychiatric Study of Terminality. New York: Human Science Press, 1972.

Whitehead, A.N. Process and Reality, corrected edition. New York: Free Press, 1979.

Death and Identity:
Implications for Pastoral Care

Gary L. Harbaugh

Although listening is always crucial in pastoral care, at
no time is it more important than in work with persons in situations of loss. I suggest that careful listening in loss situations such as terminal illness or bereavement alerts the pastor
to a special world view maintained by the dying and the grieving. It is important to understand this view if adequate and
appropriate care is to be provided. Of course, any change in
people's way of viewing the world involves a change in their
views of themselves. Those who have observed that a loss
situation precipitates an identity crisis have helped us understand the importance of a supportive pastoral ministry during
this time of identity diffusion. I will offer a perspective on
the dynamics of this identity crisis and will suggest some implications for pastoral care.

THE WORLD OF THE DYING

My sensitivity to the special language and world view
of those in death situations was first heightened during my
doctoral work with Elisabeth Kübler-Ross at the University
of Chicago in the late 1960s. Since that time, I have encountered, in secular as well as pastoral settings, a tendency
for people who are experiencing any major loss to feel that
their world has fallen apart. Effective pastoral care in a
crisis situation, therefore, depends on the willingness of the
pastor to enter into this broken world. Even more, pastoral
care requires a willingness to remain with the pain of that
world long enough to understand it. It is important for pastors to remember that the promise of presence is not to those
who run, but to those who walk through the valley of the
shadow of death.

My experience confirms that any crisis is a loss situation, a "little d" death. However, even though situations such as divorce and physical disability could be appropriate illustrations, I prefer to discuss the world of the dying from the perspective of those who were my first teachers, those who were facing death with a capital "D." The terminally ill speak best for themselves. From their own words, we can construct a paradigm of their world (Harbaugh 1968).

At the heart of that world is the physical body. The bodily reality is the ever-present point of reference. Asked how they became ill, it is not unusual for people to respond, "That's what I'm wondering, how it got into my body!" Especially in the case of malignancy, people have the feeling of destructive invasion by an alien presence (Eissler 1970). However, coronary patients also feel that they have been physically hit, knocked down, brought low. The world has ceased to be a safe place to live in. It is hard to trust that everything will work out all right. Research has indicated that, more than the healthy, the dying focus on the physical self (Harbaugh 1969). One consequence of that focus is the initial collapse of the world of the dying. Upon hospitalization, what was a world of life and vitality becomes a ward, a room, a body. Since the threat is initially perceived as a physical threat, it is small wonder that patients first articulate "help" in terms of physical intervention, and associate "health" with bodily well-being rather than with their wholeness as persons. The pastor needs to understand that, in a loss situation, the world has been radically reduced to the concrete, specific, here-and-now physical realities of life. This is why early crisis intervention is not a time for pastoral proclamation, but for pastoral presence. The most fitting word may well be the physical touch that reaches into that collapsed world and says that the person is not alone.

No matter how immediate the physical dimension, people are, of course, more than their bodies. Like those in any loss situation, the terminally ill have a real need to put what is happening to them into some kind of interpretive framework. The families of critically ill people experience the same quest for meaning. Some will speak of "God's will," which represents their attempt to understand. However, the doubt that shadows this searching is evident in the question that frequently follows the affirmation of faith, "I can't believe that God is anything less than wise, merciful, loving . . . but why me?"

There seems to be a correlation between the way individuals perceive the meaning of dying and their feelings about the meaning of living. For many, the meaning of life has been related to meaningful roles. The young woman whose life is centered in her motherhood may somewhat guiltily say she is "afraid now of who is taking care of my family. I feel that

I'm the one responsible--so much responsible--and I can do so little now." The achievement-oriented, middle-aged executive for whom life means work says, "As long as I function, I live." The young man who has never quite gained emancipation from his parents, and who therefore struggles with more than leukemia, may protest: "The thing will blast me, and I'm not about to be blasted . . . What I want most out of life is to become a man!" For most people, the situation of terminality concentrates their attention on what is most important to them.

Pastors wisely realize that in major-loss situations, all people experience at least partial collapse of their understanding of life's meaning. The sensitive care-giver understands how important it is, under those circumstances, to be a nonjudgmental listener. The temptation is for the pastor to provide an interpretation of why the illness or accident or event occurred. Since the way one sees a "little d" or "big D" death experience is related to the way one sees life, it is very risky to offer any interpretation of a loss before one really understands what that loss means to the person who has sustained it. Pastors often feel called upon to provide an answer. The risk in "wrapping things up" theologically is that we may not have fully comprehended the question.

This leads to consideration of another dimension of the world of the dying, the emotional dimension. When the quest for meaning is not understood or is prematurely closed, the person who has experienced a loss feels very much isolated: "Why in the world can't they talk to me. . . . I'm all alone." Kübler-Ross (1969) pointed out how desperately the dying need dialogue, particularly as they experience the confusing and sometimes overwhelming emotional response of anxiety and anger. "No, not me!" "I hate it! I have things to do. I wish I hadn't gotten sick." Reactive depression may lead to despair: "You come to the realization that maybe you won't ever get well. You get disgusted. . . . Life has no meaning." Although acceptance is possible, it is by no means inevitable; frequently, instead of acceptance, there is resignation, "I'm very tired."

So much has been written about the stages of emotion experienced by the dying that little more need be at this time except to affirm that these stages are common in any crisis experience, and to caution that every reaction to loss is, to some extent, idiosyncratic, depending on the individual's previous history and present life situation. Pastors who enter the world of one who is dying find that world populated with "voices" from that person's past that inhibit or give permission for emotional expression. Pastors can be most helpful if they are willing to hear what needs to be said without judgment and without taking misdirected anger as if it were a personal attack. Care also requires that pastors not expect persons to react as they would hope or like them to. Many extrinsically religious persons never reach acceptance, whereas those without religious commitment sometimes appear able to affirm their lives within the context of loss. Those who have accepted life seem the better equipped to accept the end of life (Elam 1969; Malino 1966).

Acceptance of life and of death involves others in significant ways. It is, for example, in interpersonal relations that the various physical, mental, and emotional concerns experienced by the dying seem to find primary expression. The stages of emotional response might even be defined in terms of moving toward or away from other persons. Those in loss situations have a real need for the presence of other people and for communication with them, as long as they can control the opening and the closing of that communication. When there have been meaningful relationships prior to the illness, these may be drawn on as a source of strength: "It helps, then, to have people with you? 'Oh, yes, especially certain people. . . . We have been able, with all our problems, to face them.'" But when there has been estrangement, the onset and progression of a terminal illness only aggravates the separation and emphasizes the isolation, "I'm all alone." Pastors need to make a reality-oriented assessment of the social support systems of those in loss situations. Of course, the pastors themselves are a vital part of those support systems.

In summary, the situation of terminal illness--and, in my opinion, any "death" experience--calls forth from the dying person a new self-awareness as a bodily being, a meaning-seeking being, and an emotional being. This focus on the self affects and effects a new self-world correlation, and is manifested most clearly in the realm of interpersonal relationships. In both the personal and interpersonal arenas, there appears to be a concentration on the essentials, a sharpening and deepening of the sense of what really is important in life. It may be that the concentration on the self that the existential situation of terminal illness seems to precipitate may be the precondition for the kind of questioning that results in a reappraisal of personal values. The search for meaning may well be stimulated by those experiences that most seriously call into question the existence of meaning. Unfortunately, the anxiety that normally accompanies adversity may be so high that it renders those who are experiencing a loss less accessible and diminishes their ability to integrate the loss meaningfully into their lives. Effective and faithful pastoral care recognizes the changes in the world view of those who are experiencing one or another form of death. The pastor enters into that world to understand it and to stand with those whose worlds are in danger of collapse and who, at the same time, have the opportunity to achieve self-world integration.

Timing is of paramount importance. Significantly, biblical Greek has two words for time: <u>chronos</u> and <u>kairos</u>. Chronos, of course, is calendar or clock time. Kairos is a special time used by the biblical writers to mark God's gracious inbreaking into the human situation, as in the Christ-event. The pastor's willingness to be present during the chronos of crisis makes it more likely that the suffering person will see the pastor as a resource when they are receptive to kairos, that in-breaking time of deeper self-world-God integration. Such integration is more possible when we appreciate the interrelationship of death and identity.

DEATH AND IDENTITY

The dynamic of death and resurrection undergirds Christian theology, and is also known in other religious understandings of life. In the situation of loss, any loss, something dies. The world is no longer the same, and the person in relation to this new world is also in the process of change. Even though the loss may not be threatening to physical life, pastors have learned that underlying the anxiety of loss situations is existential anxiety, as loss is always related to death.

In terms of practical implications for ministry, however, pastors have often had difficulty reconciling various views of death. Existential philosophers and psychologists have helpfully focused attention on death. However, in their focus on the person in the situation, existentialists have tended to overlook the importance of the individual's history (Gray 1967). Pastoral care-givers who are willing to enter the world of a dying person know that an appreciation of that person's history is essential to the provision of care that is adequate as well as appropriate.

Developmental psychologists, on the other hand, have accentuated individual history to such an extent that they have reduced existential fear of death to nothing but separation or castration anxiety (Freud 1962; Sarnoff and Corwin 1959). The caring pastor is unable to dismiss a parishioner's struggle for life and meaning as nothing more than the reappearance of a childhood conflict.

The pastoral theologian is concerned with integration of the developmental and the existential in order to minister to the whole person in relationship to God. The situation of loss provides an opportunity for us to explore the dynamics of the identity crisis precipitated by a death experience, and to suggest some implications for pastoral care. In my opinion, developmental and existential considerations are brought together in the boundary situation of death. A death situation inevitably raises the question of the meaning of history, or at least the meaning of the personal history of the sufferer.

Most pastors trained in recent years have been introduced, through the developmental psychology of Erikson, to
at least one way of conceptualizing individual history. Erikson
(1959a, 1964) identified eight stages of development, each involving a psychosocial crisis. These crises can be successfully resolved by favorable interaction and mutual regulation
of the individual and the nurturing or social environment.
Erikson's developmental scheme as a whole emphasizes identity, but the stage-specific crises are defined as basic trust
vs. mistrust, autonomy vs. shame and doubt, initiative vs.
guilt, industry vs. inferiority, identity vs. identity diffusion,
intimacy vs. isolation, generativity vs. stagnation, and integrity vs. despair.

As noted earlier, the dying express their thoughts and
feelings about their situation in many ways, verbal and non-
verbal. While listening to the dying, we noted such thought-
feelings as: "That's what I'm wondering, how it got into my body";
"I can't believe that God is anything less than wise . . . but why
me?"; "I feel that I'm the one responsible--so much responsible";
"I can do so little now"; "What I want most out of life is to become a man"; "Why in the world can't they talk to me . . . I'm all
alone"; "As long as I function, I live"; "You come to the realization that maybe you won't ever get well"; "I hate it!"; You get
disgusted"; "Life has no meaning."

A perceptive listener is struck by the correspondence
of so many of the verbalizations of the terminally ill with the
negative poles of Erikson's (1959, 1964) eight life-stage polar-
ities: basic mistrust, shame and doubt, guilt, inferiority,
identity diffusion, isolation, stagnation, despair. In the clinical situation, we noted a concentration on the essentials, a
sharpening and deepening of the sense of what is really important in life, a search for meaning in precisely those experiences that most seriously call into question the experience
of meaning. Erikson (1958, 1959) discussed many of these
considerations in relation to his concept of identity crisis.

The correspondence between the foci of the terminally
ill and Erikson's emphases leads me to suggest that at the
prospect of death, people recapitulate their developmental
crises in a final identity crisis, a struggling quest for coher-
ence, wholeness, and completeness--theologically, for salvation. My reading of Erikson is that each of the eight nuclear
conflicts arises, meets its crisis, and resolves during the
stage indicated. But all of the conflicts exist from the beginning in some form, and "every act calls for an integration of
all" (Harbaugh 1973). An unstated but clear corollary of this
concept is that the act of dying also calls for an integration
of the nuclear conflicts. I believe that my notion of recapitulation in the face of impending death is dynamically true and
formally complementary to Erikson's emphases, inasmuch as
death frequently appears much earlier in the life cycle than

Erikson's final stage of ego integrity vs. despair. Further-more, the accent on identity is consistent with Erikson's per-vasive orientation toward the pivotal importance of identity in all human experience.

IMPLICATIONS FOR PASTORAL CARE

Earlier we noted that those who seem best able to af-firm their lives in the face of death are those who have worked through the crises of living. That is, the way one has been engaged in life bears heavily on one's encounter with death. This clinical observation is consistent with Erik-son's description of the implications of facing death with ego integrity. It is also consonant with my contention that the existential and the developmental are integrated into the ex-perience of the terminally ill. If terminal illness (or other significant loss situation) elicits both a recapitulation of life-cycle crises and an integration of the historical and the ex-istential, then this has important implications for pastoral care. First, pastors will not be at all surprised to hear those who are terminally ill express mistrust, shame and doubt, guilt, feelings of inferiority, isolation, stagnation, and de-spair. The pastor will understand that these feelings may acquire special intensity and urgency as those people strug-gle with a situation that threatens the core of personal iden-tity.

Second, pastors will be aware of the importance of hearing each person's story, including childhood remembranc-es involving trust and autonomy, understanding that earlier resolutions of developmental crises render a person more or less adequate to face death or other major loss.

Third, pastors will develop a renewed appreciation for the ministry of the laity in providing care to those in loss situations. Erikson's work supports a relational theology, which emphasizes the interrelationship of personhood and the experience of communion with others. In interpersonal rela-tionships, there is the potential for the keenest pain, but also for the truest sense of being upheld and enabled to live life fully into death. As in the life-cycle, one is drawn into personhood by engagement with other persons. The presence of those who care enough to be there, to listen, to share, to speak when it is time for speaking and to be silent when the touch of a hand means more than words is the essence of the gift and response that reaffirms the dying parishioner as a person with all the greatness and dignity of personhood.

Fourth, in pastors' own interactions with those who are experiencing the death or other loss, they will be informed about how best to help them to deepen personal integration of the existential situation. In addition to making an intentional

effort to assist them to express their negative feelings within
the framework of acceptance and love, pastors, mindful of
Erikson's framework, will recognize that no further theological integration will be likely without the establishment of trust
between themselves and these parishioners. Pastoral presence
redevelops the parishioners' trust that they are not alone.
Active listening, emphasizing reflective responses, is essential, for it usually conveys the listener's desire to understand
what the world looks and feels like to the one who speaks.
Such fundamentals as eye contact, congruence of words and
body language, and the avoidance of either overoptimism or
undue pessimism contribute to the building of a climate of
trust.

In a crisis, people normally regress to a somewhat more
dependent stage. Pastors who know that the developmental
and existential are integrated in situations of loss will recognize the need for dependency and will assist people in areas
where assistance is needed, but will do nothing for them that
they can do for themselves. Kübler-Ross's (1969) stage of
anger has much to do with this loss of control and autonomy.
Along with the need to express their feelings, people in loss
situations need to reestablish whatever reasonable and realistic control is possible. Even when these people are bedfast
and able to do little but speak, it is usually possible for them
to participate in setting the time of the pastor's next visit.
For example, the pastor may say: "I want to stop and see
you tomorrow. Would you like me to come in the morning or
in the afternoon?" An appreciation for the recapitulation of
autonomy vs. shame and doubt will sensitize pastors to the
need to provide opportunities for people in the loss situations
to ventilate the feelings that accompany the negative pole
(shame and doubt) and to be reinforced in the regaining of
as much autonomy and control as possible.

This basic approach holds for the remaining recapitulated life-cycle stages. From the stage of initiative vs. guilt,
pastors learn to listen for indications of unfinished business
in the area of initiative--those actions taken and those not
taken (commission and omission). These may represent areas
of guilt which, at the appropriate time, may be addressed
sacramentally or through private confession and absolution.
Other Eriksonian stages alert pastors to the possibility that
those in loss situations have linked performance and achievement with personal identity and personal acceptability. Since
most people in crisis are not able to function normally, they
may feel powerless, worthless, and unacceptable. If condition-
al acceptance is equated with love, they may feel in danger
of losing love when they can no longer meet the "conditions."
Thus, pastors may find it important to help the parishioners
express these feelings, which are symptomatic of depression,
and then help them see what they still have to give to their

significant others, including the opportunity to deal openly and honestly with what is happening in their lives. Such efforts can also help offset the sense of isolation that most people feel in crisis situations.

Erikson's final stage of integrity vs. despair requires special attention. In her seminal work, Kübler-Ross (1969) discussed the final stage of acceptance, which comes only when a loss has been worked through. Kübler-Ross differentiates acceptance from resignation, which represents a giving in without a working through of the earlier stages of death. In contrast, acceptance is a "yes" to life. This is consistent with the view expressed by Erikson, who also speaks of integrity as looking back over "one's one and only life-cycle," and affirming it. In Christian theology, the courage to say "yes" to life in the face of death and to say "yes" to death in the midst of life is grounded in the gift of God's "yes" to us in Christ. Just as it is necessary in human development to "die" to one stage of life in order to be "born" into another, so people of faith face death with trust and hope. The final stage of integrity, then, is linked to the first stage of trust.

Ministry in loss situations is a ministry of presence that reestablishes trust and represents hope. Through careful listening, pastors are able to be present and even to enter, insofar as it is possible, into the collapsed "world of the dying." Sensitivity to that world in terms of sufferers' restructuring of the physical, mental, emotional, and social dimensions of their humanness can help pastors make appropriate responses. When a major loss is perceived as precipitating an identity crisis in which the life-cycle crises are recapitulated, pastoral ministry not only becomes more appropriate, but also more adequate. The promise of presence even in the valley of the shadow of death is fulfilled through the presence of pastoral people, ordained and lay, who incarnate the trustworthiness of that promise.

REFERENCES

Eissler, K.R. The Psychiatrist and the Dying Patient, p. 167. New York: International Universities Press, 1970.

Elam, L.C. "A Psychiatric Perspective on Death." In L.O. Mills, ed., Perspectives on Death, p. 203. New York: Abingdon Press, 1969.

Erikson, E.H. Young Man Luther. A Study in Psychoanalysis and History, Austen Riggs Center Monograph No. 4, pp. 99-104, 113-115, 170-222, 160ff. New York: W.W. Norton, 1958.

---. "Growth and Crisis of the Healthy Personality." Psychological Issues. Monograph, vol. 1, no. 1, pp. 88-94,
101-164. New York: International Universities Press,
1959a.

---. "Identity and the Life Cycle." Psychological Issues.
Monograph, vol. 2, no. 1, pp. 50-100. New York:
International Universities Press, 1959b.

---. Childhood and Society. New York: W.W. Norton, 1964.

Freud, S. The Ego and the Id, Standard Edition, p. 87.
Translated by J. Riviere. New York: W.W. Norton,
1962.

Gray, J.G. "The Problem of Death in Modern Philosophy." In
N. Scott, ed., The Modern Vision of Death. Richmond,
Va.: John Knox Press, 1967.

Harbaugh, G.L. "The Voice of the Dying." Unpublished dissertation, University of Chicago, 1968.

---. "Perceptual and Value Differences Between the Terminally Ill and the Physically Healthy." University of
Chicago, 1969.

---. "Death: A Theological Reformulation of Developmental
and Existential Perspectives." Unpublished dissertation,
University of Chicago, 1973.

Kübler-Ross, E. On Death and Dying. New York: Macmillan,
1969.

Malino, J.R. "Coping with Death in Western Religious Civilization." Zygon: Journal of Religion and Science 1:4
(1966), 364.

Sarnoff, I. and S.M. Corwin. "Castration Anxiety and the
Fear of Death." Journal of Personality 27 (1959), 374-
385.

4

Issues Facing Clergy on the Hospice Team

Virginia A. Samuel

Encounters with staff, patients, and families during three years' work as a hospice chaplain have left me profoundly changed. I have grown in my desire to live life to the fullest and in ability to establish priorities in the relationships and activities of my life. This growth did not come automatically, but slowly, with great pain and difficulty. It came only as I took time to reflect about myself and my internal life. With that self-reflection, I was able to see the changes taking place and to claim for myself the growing I was doing.

It is essential for people in any helping profession to be in touch with their own feelings and thoughts, hopes, and dreams. Perhaps this is especially true for those who work with dying people and their families because, by its nature, this work can be physically, emotionally, and spiritually draining. Not to know oneself is to risk becoming burned out without even realizing it. When that happens, it not only compromises one's ability to minister effectively to patients and their families, but also risks harm to oneself.

It is my hope that what I write here will be of help to others in their ministries; it is not meant to be exhaustive, but to raise some pastoral care issues that confront clergy who work in hospices. These facilities, which provide care for dying people and their families, are staffed by interdisciplinary teams that include doctors, nurses, social workers, chaplains, program coordinators, and volunteers. In effect, the hospice chaplain is in team ministry. Several issues arise when chaplains work directly with patients and families and as part of a team. Many of the same issues arise for the other team members as well but, for the purposes of this chapter, I will refer primarily to chaplains.

One issue that comes up frequently concerns the legitimacy of the chaplain's position on the team. The chaplain's role is recognized as an important one by the National Hospice Organization. Nevertheless, that recognition alone does not guarantee that chaplains will feel that they belong.

In our culture, doctors are seen as the ones best qualified to make decisions about patient care. They are usually seen as the only ones who have the knowledge and skill to bring about physical healing. Less emphasis is put on the spiritual and emotional healing needed by people faced with illness. Consequently, the clergy have historically been called to visit patients when doctors can do no more to effect a physical cure.

Hospice challenges that traditional model of medical care by viewing each member of the team, including the chaplain, as having equal weight in recommending care plans. However, unless chaplains have a good sense of their own authority, are convinced of the vital importance of the patient's spiritual health, and feel strongly about their own ability to address that health, they will be reluctant to speak up about profound spiritual issues during patient-review meetings. Consequently, not only will other team members remain uninformed about spiritual issues, but those issues will not be addressed in the team's care of patients and their families.

Chaplains' reluctance to be assertive about their role may come from another source as well, namely their own uncertainty about what spiritual issues are. By "spiritual issues," I mean those that are concerned with the quality of people's lives and the meaning, or lack of it, in their relationships with God, others, and themselves. Spiritual issues have to do with people's desire to live or to die, and the reasons for those feelings. They have to do with people's values and how they plan to spend the time they have left to live on earth. Hospice chaplains should be able to make spiritual diagnoses of patients, family members, and even staff members. They should be able to articulate clearly the spiritual issues that arise in particular cases.

Another problem for hospice chaplains is their ability to function as part of a team. Clergy have often been seen as people who prefer to work alone. "The Lone Ranger" is a name frequently given to clergy who act as if they are the only ones able to perform certain tasks, and who do not seek the help and cooperation of others as often as they might. Membership on a hospice team calls for something quite different. It requires each team member to have a commitment to cooperate with the others and to have a sense of striving toward a common goal. Although each discipline has its own particular area of expertise, each team member must have a genuine respect for the other disciplines. Such respect facilitates group sharing about each patient or family situation and

encourages all involved to offer opinions about the patient-
care plan.

The hospice chaplain must be respectful of other team
members' views. That means, in part, listening to their
views of the spiritual issues involved in any case. It also
means that chaplains should encourage the others to make
spiritual diagnoses of situations and to deal with the emotional and spiritual concerns of patients and family members.
Such action by chaplains not only fosters a feeling of team-
work, but also helps reduce the possibility that other team
members will feel uncomfortable in dealing with spiritual issues. When someone asks, "Would you like to see our chaplain?", it can be a way of cutting off discussion by communicating the message that "I don't deal with that concern, the
chaplain does." If team members are cognizant of and comfortable with spiritual issues and are encouraged to deal with
them as they arise, the number of "missed chances," times
when patients or family members are ready to talk but no one
is ready to listen, will be lessened. For this to happen, the
chaplain must be committed to being a team member.

A third concern has to do with pastoral care of the
team. It is inevitable that team members will become emotionally involved with patients and family members. However, if
a team member consistently does not feel anything, that may
be a sign of burnout. The shutting down of feelings is a defense. The nature of hospice work involves a process of con-
tinual grieving. The chaplain must be aware of this, aware
of the dynamics of grief, and aware of the unique way each
team member grieves. The chaplain must encourage them to
express their grief in appropriate ways. Pastoral care of the
hospice team is just as important as pastoral care of patients
and their families.

The chaplain is also involved in constant grief work,
and therefore is also in need of pastoral care. Chaplains who
are reluctant to allow others on the team to care for them in
this way not only risk harm to themselves, but also foster a
breakdown in the team spirit. A caring relationship is a two-
way street, calling for all team members to give and receive
pastoral care as needed. The ability of chaplains to admit
their own pain, grief, fears, and hopes, to express them in
appropriate ways, and to receive support from other team
members is crucial to the health of the team. Modeling self-
care by expressing one's feelings and allowing others to make
caring responses is one way to help other team members take
better care of themselves in the same way.

The chaplain must also be attentive to issues that arise
from interaction with patients and their family members. In
ministering to dying people, chaplains confront death in a
dramatic way. In the process, they are confronted with the

way they view death and their feelings about it. It is essential that people who serve as hospice chaplains be willing to
be in touch with and explore their feelings about their own
death and the deaths of others, about past losses and griefs,
and about pain and suffering. Chaplains' unknown feelings
about death will control and contaminate their interactions
with patients, families, and hospice staff. Knowing themselves
enables chaplains to put aside their own conscious or unconscious need to work out their unresolved feelings and grief.
It also enables them to put aside their need for people to die
the "good death," and allows them to allow patients to confront death in their own unique ways and to die as they will.

Chaplains must also be in touch with their own limits.
Hospice work is both fulfilling and draining. It is important
for chaplains to be aware of the limits of their caring,
strength, and willingness to be involved, and to accept
those limits as safeguards against burnout. Further, it is essential for chaplains to find ways to disengage temporarily
from their emotion-laden work so that they can maintain their
equilibrium and be emotionally and spiritually restored. Ideal-
ly, chaplains monitor themselves constantly and take care of
themselves in such a way that burnout does not happen because of a backlog of feelings that were not taken seriously.

For dying people in our culture, often one of the most
painful parts of the process is a feeling of isolation. We are,
generally speaking, a death-denying culture. We go to great
lengths, not only to deny the inevitability of death, but the
fact of death once it has occurred. A quick look at our
youth-worshiping media and our funeral practices, in which
the body is made to look as lifelike as possible, confirms this.
One result of these attitudes is that we have become a people
who are uncomfortable in the face of death and who do not
know what to say to someone experiencing it firsthand. Consequently, several things may happen, and often do. Friends
and family may fail to visit the person who is dying. The
patient is then alone as contact with the outside world dwin-
dles.

Another form of isolation that occurs frequently is
harder to understand because it does not reflect the external
situation. This is the isolation that arises when those who
visit patients or family members do not allow them to express
their feelings about what's going on. Discussions about the
weather, the doctor's good reports, the improved appearance
of the patient, and similar feeling-denying approaches isolate
patients and their family members. These approaches quietly
but powerfully convey to patients the following message:
"Tell me you are feeling better. Tell me you will be getting
well and that you are not going to die." To family members,
the message is "I can't bear hearing about your breaking
heart. It isn't true, your loved one will get better." Although

such statements may help the visitor to feel better, they rarely do so for the patients or families. Usually, they are left feeling that no one cares, that they must live a lie and put up a good front, and that to show their true state, involving very powerful, painful feelings, is unacceptable. This lack of acceptance quickly leads to feelings of isolation which, in themselves, are painful.

In such situations, one of the most important and valuable things hospice chaplains can do is to listen to patients and family members and encourage them to express the intense feelings surrounding the situation. Effective listening involves hearing both the expressed and unexpressed feelings. Hospice chaplains must be able to hear the feelings behind the words of patients and their family members and to explore with them the meaning of their words and the feelings that underlie them. Another name for such listening is "active listening." As chaplains listen in this way and convey willingness to enter into the speaker's experience, as unpleasant as it is, the speaker will begin to feel valued and valuable, accepted and acceptable, less isolated and alone.

This willingness of chaplains to put self aside and to enter the other's world is called "presence." In and of itself, it is a healing thing. Clergy who work with hospices must be convinced of that fact. Those who are not will spend their time trying to "do something" to alter the externals of the situation. That is to miss the point entirely. There is often nothing that we can do to change the external situation. Besides that, the internal lives of patients and their families are the primary concern of chaplains. By listening, caring, and being present to others, chaplains can help them to muster their own particular strengths to face the situation and change the internal lives of patients and family members. "Nothing has changed, but I feel better" is a frequent statement made by those who have benefited by the "presence" of a chaplain.

Once chaplains are listening attentively, they should expect to hear and be prepared to deal with the powerful emotions that may be expressed. Feelings of being overwhelmed, of anger, sadness, despair, hopelessness, helplessness, and anxiety are quite common in hospice families. Feelings of joy, relief, and hope are also experienced as patients and families cling to each sign of improvement and each positive report from the doctor. All of these feelings are apt to be intensified in light of the impending death and separation. Individuals will often feel as though they are going crazy because their feelings seem overwhelming and unmanageable.

A woman whose sister was dying told me: "Fear clouds over everything. It robs me of my strength, robs me even of the knowledge that I have strength. I feel like a child--I just want somebody to fix it. I feel like a baby bird in a nest

with somebody shaking the tree." My response was to listen
to the woman, encourage her to tell me more about her fears,
and not to try to talk her out of her feelings. As a result,
she was finally able to affirm for herself that she was not going crazy, and that although she was afraid, she would not
be destroyed by the fear.

In this situation, I was also able to convey to this woman, by nonjudgmental listening and by my presence, that she
was acceptable. My faith in her helped her to have faith in
herself and in her ability to handle the situation. At one point
in our conversation, I expressed faith that God would be with
her and would give her what she needed to face her sister's
death. She replied: "I believe that, but I need to hear more
about your belief in me. It's myself I doubt, not God." I responded by sharing my conviction that I did have faith in her
ability to be with her sister while she died and then to survive the loss of that relationship.

People who are facing death usually spend some time
reviewing the quality of their lives. Frequently, they become
acutely aware of the shortcomings and failures in their relationships to God, others, and themselves. As they become
aware of the guilt and regret they feel, they need someone to
whom they can confess their shortcomings and through whom
God's grace and forgiveness can be mediated. This is a very
important part of the chaplain's job in a hospice. Confession
and absolution are very real needs of dying people.

Some traditions have specific rites and rituals for confession and absolution; others do not. The important thing is
that chaplains be aware that the process of confession is an
important one for the dying person. They must be prepared
to hear the person's confession and to offer absolution at the
appropriate time.

Family members frequently need to confess the hurts
and regrets they feel in relation to the dying person. It is
important for chaplains to facilitate conversation between patients and family members along these lines. Often reconciliation between the patient and family comes first, and then,
together, they are reconciled with God. Often these events
occur in reverse order. I think the order is less important
than the fact that both occur. A very important part of the
chaplain's job is to facilitate forgiveness and reconciliation,
and to convey God's grace in as many ways as possible.

Dying is a painful process emotionally, spiritually, and
often physically. Watching a loved one die is painful. Often
life loses its meaning for all involved. It becomes a mechani-
cal, routine series of days empty of the joy and vitality it
once held. As relationships draw to a close, through no choice
of the people involved, and as people realize that the plans and
dreams they had together will not come to pass, hope often
ebbs. Humans cannot live without hope, and yet dying people

and their families often feel as if there is no hope for them.
One of the most important parts of the chaplain's job is to
offer hope.

When most patients and family members think of hoping
for something, they hope for a reversal of the dying process
and the patient's restoration to perfect health. In some cases,
that is realistic, and the chaplain can join in support. In
other situations, however, the patient will not recover, and
hope for that outcome is not realistic. Knowing when to encourage that hope and when to point out to the people involved that it is unrealistic requires that the chaplain be extremely sensitive and work in close contact with the other members
of the hospice team. I believe it is important not to break
through people's defenses deliberately, but to offer a combination of gentle confrontation and support of individuals' hopes
and denial when they clearly need them.

Apart from the hope of physical cure, there is much
hope that chaplains can offer. Relief from pain, reconciliation
with others, and a better day tomorrow are all legitimate,
healing hopes that chaplains can offer to patients and family
members alike. Above all, chaplains should convey in as many
ways as possible the thought that God is present, that He
knows and cares about the patient and the family, that He for-
gives all that is past, and that He will sustain them through
the moment of death and beyond. I have seen people visibly
relieved and relaxed when we have talked about God and together have expressed these hopes.

Chaplains should know their own tradition's particular
resources of faith and be comfortable offering them at appropriate times. When chaplains are called to families whose tradition is different from their own, they should be willing to
explore the resources of that tradition and discover what has
meaning for this family. An ecumenical spirit and a willingness
to mediate other traditions when possible are essential char-
acteristics of hospice chaplains.

One particular prayer has frequently helped me to minister to patients and family members:

> Lord, grant me the serenity
> to accept the things I cannot change,
> the courage to change the things I can,
> and the wisdom to know the difference.

The Serenity Prayer helped me a great deal to be realistic about what I could and couldn't do for others and to
content myself with what I did have to offer to help them in
Christ's name. It is my hope that clergy seeking to minister
to those who are about to leave this life and those who love
them will be filled with God's grace, love, and forgiveness
and be able to convey that to them. They will be blessed in
the process.

5

"The Flower Fadeth"—
A Pastoral-Care Curriculum for Biblical
Death Education in the Church

Jeffrey A. Watson

In the past 15 years there has been a contagious explo-
sion of interest in the topic of death and dying. This avid
curiosity has been present on both the popular and professional levels. Resulting from this quest for the understanding of
death, a new discipline has arisen. It is called thanatology.
In partnership with this discipline, professional societies have
been formed, journals produced, research literature published,
symposia offered, and auxilliary institutions begun.[1] It is imperative that the institutional church consider significant involvement in this movement.

Research in thanatology to date has focused on individual patient concerns.[2] However, considerable research has
also been devoted to theoretical issues[3] and to interventional
techniques.[4] It is only in the most recent years that the implications of the foregoing research have sponsored mature
proposals for institutional modifications.[5] It is at this juncture
that the church must project itself as a relevant and contemporary institution within the society.

THE NEED FOR BIBLICAL DEATH
EDUCATION IN THE CHURCH

The unique needs of the aged, dying, and bereaved
person require appropriate spiritual care. The average leader

---

This curriculum design represents an expansion and
revision of an earlier monograph: Jeffrey A. Watson, "Death
Education in the Church: An Instrument of Pastoral Care for
the Dying and Bereaved." It was written and simultaneously
presented as a seminar paper to fellow students in the doctor-

and member in the church feel somewhat unprepared to offer this kind of spiritual care. It is therefore imperative that the church offer holistic biblical death education to its leaders and its members so that these unique needs can be understood and met as they arise.

When a person has a medical diagnosis that projects life expectancy to be less than six months, he or she is usually classified as terminally ill. This diagnosis generally applies to people with chronic degenerative diseases. After a person has received such a diagnosis, his or her spiritual and emotional needs may become just as acute as physical needs. This person begins to wrestle with the reality of impending death. Similarly, the acutely aged or recently bereaved person is often placed in a comparable crisis with his or her own confrontation with death. These months or years of crisis for the person surrounded by death provide a unique and significant opportunity for Christian ministry.

Holism

When Paul blessed the believers at Thessalonica, he prayed for God's special grace on their ". . . spirit and soul and body . . . unto the coming of our Lord Jesus Christ."[6] He saw an interdependence between the spiritual, emotional, and physical needs of the whole person. This same interconnection between spiritual well-being and general health is clearly made elsewhere in the Scriptures as well.[7] It is interesting that even in our culture we have holistic derivatives from our old English word halus. This one word exists today as "whole, holy, and health."[8] Again there is a thematic connection between spiritual well-being, general healthiness, and to being whole.

Our Lord was concerned to meet needs on every level of human existence. He healed blindness, befriended the social outcast, and preached about being born again into an unearthly kingdom. He did not ignore physical needs or minimalize emotional pain. Most of all He could not pretend that the deep spiritual needs of man were unimportant. Metaphysical reality was never to be diluted by infatuation with the material world.[9] When the Lord commended those who would "visit the sick" (Matt. 25:36), He described their visiting ministry with the Greek word spiskope ("to inspect, to look over diligently, to oversee"). Epperly amplifies the concept

---

of course, "The Philosophy and Practice of Ministry" (Dallas, Tex.: Dallas Theological Seminary, 1982). This curriculum design represents a detailed expansion and modification of the earlier monograph.

by saying, "The gist of the word implies a vision of the person which involves an overarching panorama of the needs of the whole person. This concept is the forerunner of the current holistic care movement."[10]

It is in Mark's gospel that the majority of Christ's physical healings are recorded. And yet even here Christ's frequent commands for the healed person not to tell anyone of the healing is significant. A commentator suggests a reason for this odd command:

> Jesus did not want the broadcast of these healings to give a distorted message that the needs of the body might be seen as transcending the need of the mind, emotions, and spirit. Rather than have this vision of man projected, he requested, to no avail, that these healings not be mentioned at all. Jesus' concern, however, has largely come true in our time as we urgently wage war against death and disease and yet casually seek to meet the needs of the spirit.[11]

In light of this holistic priority, physicians must avoid "playing God" in the medical arena.[12] Health-care professionals must assess the whole person.[13] Training institutions must equip people-helpers with a broader range of skills for healing.[14] And foremost, spiritual-care providers must not underestimate their role in the health-care process.

> Spiritual care is more than a nice "extra," it is a vital ingredient in health care. Each person is a biologically, psychosocially, and spiritually integrated being, created to live in relationship with other people and with God. Illness disrupts the harmony of that integration and often alters relationships with others and with God. I doubt that anyone would question the inter-relationship between the biological and psychosocial dimensions of a person, but many health care providers simply overlook the spiritual dimension. . . . Spiritual care is an integrating factor in health care. Respecting and encouraging a person's spiritual and religious interests and concerns enhances the healing process. Spiritual support includes communicating love, forgiveness, meaning, purpose and hope in a time of discouragement and anxiety. It is not a frill. It is basic to good health care.[15]

The Needs of the Dying, the Aged,
and the Bereaved

The dying person has some unique needs. Apart from
the biomedical crisis, he or she is unusually prone to anxiety
and depression.[16] Despair, feelings of helplessness, and
social isolation are often the most painful aspects of dying.
It becomes imperative that the family and support team tend to
the patient's psychological well-being[17] as well as spiritual
needs.[18] Regardless of where the dying person is located--
hospital, nursing home, clinical hospice, or family home--he
or she has several universal needs. These are physical care,
relief of symptoms, independence, dignity, and acceptance by
others of one's individual approach to dying.[19] A Christian
nurse in a religious hospital summarizes her concept of care
for a dying person.

> Assuming, then, that the patient is going to
> die, our duty then becomes one of preparing the
> patient to die in a way that benefits one of God's
> creatures about to face his own particular judg-
> ment and to enter into eternal life, and all treat-
> ment should be benefit to the patient, to help
> him live as fully as possible until he dies, so
> providing the opportunity to prepare for death.
> This true conception of death is one that comes
> naturally to us as Christians . . .[20]

After the medical destiny of the dying person has become apparent, the model of helping must shift from curing
to caring. The care-givers must move away from trying to
change the dying person's destiny and begin helping him or
her cope with the massive adjustments to dying.[21] Professionals, volunteers, and family must come to appreciate the enor-
mous physical, psychological, and spiritual components of the
patient's pain.[22] People who do involve themselves with dying
family members and who witness the values of palliative care
usually resolve their grief more effectively.[23] Likewise, spiritual-care providers who move away from a merely curative
agenda are able to offer a more thorough ministry to the dying person and the family.[24]
Irrespective of health problems, the elderly person is
more anxious about afterlife.[25] He or she experiences unique
psychological needs,[26] death anxieties,[27] and problems with
aging.[28] The spiritual care of the aged person should seek to
provide healthy relationships,[29] community orientation,[30] and
relevant instruction.[31] Those who offer Christian ministry to
the elderly should take note of any sudden interest or loss
of interest in religion by the older person. This is sometimes
an early warning signal of suicidal thoughts.[32] In general,

research supports an open invitation among the elderly for
religious ministry.[33] Such an opportunity must not be ignored
by family and spiritual-care providers.

It will be important to the aged that their care-providers
emphasize "living" over "dying." While it is obvious that dying will happen to all of us and may appear to be happening
faster with the aged, they are still alive. We must never
lapse into a stereotype of the aged where we presume that
their life-filled activities and emotion-filled memories are not
pulsating with vitality. While the elderly are sometimes pre-
judged to be rigid or inflexible, it is often the younger relative or care-provider who fits that description better. It is
often the younger person who presumes that he or she must
be the helper. It is often the younger person who presumes
that there is no life in a quiet view from a window, in a
repeated story, in a simple drive to a familiar place, in a
friendly conversation, in a leisurely walk, in a senior romance,
in a child's face, or in a plain task. Let the younger person
learn from and benefit by the older person. Let him or her
learn to recognize life when he sees it. Let both the young
and the old learn to live in light of reality and enrich the
lives of one another.

The Role of Spiritual Care-Providers

Clergy and lay care-givers occupy an essential role in
spiritual ministry to the sick. Some of these care-givers fulfill their role exceptionally well while others offer clearly
substandard care.[34] When a family is struggling with the realities of life and death, their needs and expectations for the
religious care-givers are extremely high.[35] The spiritual care-
provider can offer comforting security through rehearsing the
familiar beliefs and worship forms of the faith.[36] The spiritual care-giver can respond supportively during sudden medical emergencies as well as the waiting times.[37] Dayringer
likens the latter role to that of a clown.

> Clowns are not the main attraction at the circus.
> They appear between the great acts and make us
> smile. They appear to be awkward and unsuc-
> cessful in their endeavors. They seem to like us
> and to be like us. They remind us with a tear
> and a smile that we share the same human weak-
> nesses. The clown must be trained for his job
> and also be creative and original. He "gets to"
> the people, not so much by his expertise or ver-
> satility, as by his humanity.[38]

Those who provide spiritual care to very sick people
should view their role in health care positively. It was a Chi-

cago minister who invited Kübler-Ross to begin her now fa-
mous psychological research with dying patients.[39] Many
other religious care-givers have been instrumental in the hospice movement.[40] Whether one provides spiritual care as an
ordained professional or a lay volunteer, the personal qualities of love are the key ingredient to effective ministry.

> Pastoral care . . . may be defined as the
> communication of God's love to persons in need.
> It is an art more than a science, a living rela-
> tionship more than a theoretical discipline, a
> perspective more than a category of work, a
> way of being more than a way of doing. The
> clergy's presence with the sick is an indicator
> of his or her love and implies and points to the
> love of God for the sick and the family.[41]

As the care-giver extends Christ's presence in his affirming and relational ministry, there is a partial antidote to
suffering being offered.

> When potentially life-threatening illness is in-
> volved and optimal needs are high, the chap-
> lain should be an integral part of the team
> using his special skills for the relief of dis-
> tress. Although medicine and especially modern
> medicine is a true science, its application is,
> and will remain, an art, an art designed for
> the relief of distress and suffering.[42]

It should never be presumed that such qualities of spiritual
care cannot be provided in part by the health-care community
itself. Writing as a minister and psychiatrist, Merrill defends
the role of religious values in medical treatment.

> A religious orientation and familiarity with what
> people believe and how they express their beliefs
> can be a valuable resource for any doctor. Skill
> in his or her profession is of course the first
> obligation for any physician or surgeon, but the
> cold, impersonal scientist is not as well equipped
> to help troubled patients as the warm, human,
> understanding believer . . . Care of the whole
> person, in his or her physical, mental, emotional,
> social, and spiritual dimensions is what is needed
> for maximum medical effectiveness.[43]

Whether one ministers spiritual care as a religious or health-
care professional, or as a lay volunteer, one must be a believer in reality beyond the material world. Kelsey concurs

with the necessity of this metaphysical world view as one
cares for the dying.

> We cannot hope to work with the dying and
> answer their questions which death poses with-
> out such an understanding [of reality beyond
> the material world]. Ministers who plan to spend
> much time with the dying need a firm and well
> grounded conviction that there is a Reality be-
> yond the material world and in which our lives
> continue after death. They need good training
> in this thinking and also a knowledge of the
> facts that give rise to this view. There is no
> substitute for this kind of worldview. No matter
> how good our intentions are or how caring our
> bedside manner is, we still need a vision of an-
> other dimension of Reality into which one steps
> at death. The lack of this vision will inevitably
> cast a pall on our relationship with the dying.[44]

In summary, the unique needs of the aged, dying, and
bereaved person require appropriate spiritual care. In order
for this kind of care to be appropriate, it must be holistic--
attending the physical, emotional, and spiritual needs of the
person. Furthermore the care must be sensitive to his or her
distinctive needs. In addition, this care must tolerate a shift
from curing to management of distress. Finally the spiritual-
care providers must present a deeply persuaded belief in
reality beyond the material world. Since the average leader
and member in the church feels somewhat unprepared to offer
this kind of spiritual care, it is imperative that the church
offer resources for holistic biblical death education.

THE PHILOSOPHY OF BIBLICAL DEATH
EDUCATION IN THE CHURCH

Since the needs of the aged, dying, and bereaved
are unique, the church should offer appropriate spiritual
care for them. In order to offer maximum spiritual care for
these people, the church should provide resources to equip
its people with holistic biblical death education.

Mobilizing the Lay Community

Clergy and lay leaders have for some time sought to
identify individual abilities within the church and to channel
them toward the corresponding special needs.[45] Is it not
reasonable for the pastor or elder who is committed to the

ministry of the dying and bereaved to seek out a core of lay workers to extend his presence and influence in this ministry?

Developing a group of lay specialists has numerous advantages. First of all, it bypasses some of the normal clergy-laity barriers.[46] Second, it invites congregational members who have experienced a death in the family to reinvest some of their energy into altruistic service.[47] Third, it fights against the congregation's classically withdrawing from people in crisis out of feelings of inadequacy. Such a loss of social support intensifies the depression in the sick person.[48] A fourth major reason for facilitating lay care-giving teams is the effect on those who are suffering. There is a stabilizing and healing effect on the sick person when religious hope and meaning are reinforced to him by the caring community of faith. Those who are coping with chronic pain are helped by reliance upon a belief system.[49] The simple religious resources of church life and prayer are seen as more helpful to the suffering person than intense emotional or religious experiences.[50] Furthermore, healing therapies are generally improved when they are supported by religious beliefs.[51]

The lay religious community can only become aware and mobilized through a coordinated program of biblical death education over several years.[52] During the preliminary phase, church leaders ought to focus on developing congregational health and crisis-prevention strategies. This foundational period can focus on matters such as family health and systems therapy, intimacy and social-support resources, stress counseling, coping with life-change events, and the promotion of healthful aging.[53]

While the church leaders engage in promoting congregational health and crisis-prevention strategies, they can also develop a deliberate rationale for offering biblical death-education resources in the church. A proposed rationale for biblical death education may be instructive. First, death is a key biblical subject. If the quantity of biblical reference suggests logical priority, then death must be a significant part of church education.

Second, death is a major developmental crisis. Churches have devoted much time to the developmental issues in marriage and parenting over the last 20 years. More recently the church has been addressing single adulthood, mid-life crisis, and divorce. It is only consistent now to speak to the issues of old age and terminal illness.

Third, death is a critical concern to the growing elderly population in our churches. Medical advances have extended life expectancy considerably. The post-World War I baby boom generation (born between 1920-30) is now marching massively into older adulthood. Their children (the post-World-War II baby boom born between 1945-55) are being confronted with the realities of aging and death by experience with their parents. These two population pockets are demanding answers for their life experiences.

Fourth, death and dying is a popular subject outside the church. Popular bookshelves, song lyrics, and movie themes illustrate the critical concern of our society regarding death. Nuclear dangers threaten modern society daily. Any topic that becomes a critical concern of our society must be reflected in the curriculum of our churches. Just as the nation's church has been brought into a dialogue on the question of human sexuality, civil rights, and social affluence, so now society is demanding answers on the subject of death.

Fifth, death education benefits a church. When a program of biblical death education is functioning in a church, there are definite benefits both to leaders and members. The minister, who is often the mediator/interpreter of technical medical information to the family and congregation, is able to engage in some preventive education. For instance, he or she can teach people the role of grief before they are thrown into acute loss. This lessens the crisis-orientation of some intervention. The leaders can correct ignorance and misconception about death on a neutral forum before the crisis itself exposes such misinformation. The key benefit of biblical death education in the church is that it will mobilize a special core of volunteers to help nurture the aged, dying, and bereaved.

Training Lay Care-Givers

The lay care-givers who emerge from the congregation for special training in their ministry to the aged, dying, and bereaved will need to be screened. They don't need to be superhuman but they do need to be emotionally and spiritually healthy. They also need to be people who have a generally good support system available to them. These qualifications are important because each care-giver will begin to share the grief of the people they help.[54] Because the care-givers are prone to emotional burnout, many experienced leaders recommend debriefing, time off, or even grief counseling after a death has occurred.[55]

This care-giving team will be trained in several technical and personal skills. Among these are some of the more important skills: communicating verbal and nonverbal support and empathy,[56] recognizing the difference between normal and pathological grief,[57] providing home-based support for the dying person and his or her grieving family,[58] communicating bad news, and facilitating good leave-taking.[59]

Using Death-Educational Principles

Basic death-educational principles emphasize human relations. Physicians who have received death education demonstrate improved self-awareness, stress management, interpersonal communication, meaningful friendships, and professional camaraderie.[60] In order to maximize benefits to dying patients, helpful death education should focus on pain control, communication, and counseling.[61]

It is important for anyone introducing death-educational resources into a new context to recognize a couple of potential limitations to their teaching. First, death education will increase anxiety in the learners. This anxiety can express itself as resistance to the training course or as personal frustration. However, research demonstrates that this increased anxiety is temporary. It usually resolves into greater awareness and skill related to death issues.[62] Another potential limitation is in the difficulty of getting affective change. Although information can be learned with small amounts of death-educational time, deeper feelings and attitudes are not usually changed short of nine class units on death education.[63] This research finding should encourage more extended biblical death-education opportunities in the church in order to facilitate attitude and life-style change.

Church leaders who want to offer some death-educational resources to their members should be encouraged. There are numerous strategies for teaching patients,[64] for teaching the elderly,[65] and for teaching people who are currently untouched by death.[66] Practical ideas, methodologies, and materials are readily available.[67]

THE PROGRAM OF BIBLICAL DEATH EDUCATION IN THE CHURCH

The curriculum base for death education in the church should be the Judeo-Christian Scriptures. While Protestant, Catholic, and Jewish canons of Scripture differ, there is a basically compatible theology of death shared by all three traditions. Anyone who is significantly involved with death education and bereavement counseling in the twentieth century United States must have a functional familiarity with biblical teachings about death. These teachings can be used to affirm and consolidate the beliefs already held by the dying or bereaved person. Furthermore, they can be used to instruct the seeker whose confrontation with death has opened him or her to spiritual matters. Each spiritual care-giver should evaluate biblical traditions in the light of modern thanatological research. This will give credibility to biblical themes. It will also allow the nurturing care-giver to present religious concepts with contemporary relevance.

CURRICULUM

It is valuable to summarize the topics of biblical thanatology with illustrative references. These topics can form content base for lessons, sermons, devotionals, and counseling sessions in a program of biblical death education.

The Practices, Customs, and Experiences Associated with Death in Old Testament Thanatology

A. The corpses of the deceased were treated with honor.
1. Affection was demonstrated publicly (Gen. 46:4, 50:1).
2. The deceased were clothed (1 Sam. 28:14).
3. The corpses were buried to avoid exposure and abuse by predators (1 Kings 14:11; Jer. 16:4, 22:19; Ezek. 29:5).
4. Decomposing corpses were ceremonially (hygienically) unclean and thus rendered those who came in contact with them unclean (Lev. 21:1-4, 22:4; Num. 19:11-16; Ezek. 43:7; Hag. 2:13).
5. Corpses were usually unembalmed and carried on an open bier (2 Sam. 3:31; 2 Kings 13:21).
6. In an Egyptian host culture, the exceptional use of embalming and a coffin was employed (Gen. 50:2-3, 26).
7. The basic frame of the person (skeleton) was most highly protected (Gen. 50:25; Exod. 13:19; Ezek. 37:11-14).

B. Survivors displayed graphic public and private mourning.
1. They tore their clothes (Gen. 37:34; 2 Sam. 1:1, 3:31, 13:31; Job 1:20).
2. They wore sackcloth (Gen. 37:34; 2 Sam. 3:31; 2 Kings 6:30; Isa. 20:2-4; Mic. 1:8).
3. Shoes were taken off (2 Sam. 15:30; Ezek. 24:17, 23; Mic. 1:8).
4. Headdress was removed (Ezek. 24:17, 23).
5. The face or beard was veiled (2 Sam. 15:30, 19:5).
6. Hands were placed on one's head as a gesture of grief (2 Sam. 13:19; Jer. 2:37).
7. Soil was placed on one's head (Josh. 7:6; 1 Sam. 4:12; Neh. 9:1; Job 2:12; Ezek. 27:30).
8. One rolled his or her head or body in the dust (Job 16:15; Mic. 1:10).
9. One sat or lay in dust or ashes (Esther 4:3; Isa. 58:5; Jer. 6:26; Ezek. 27:30).
10. One refrained from using perfumes or soaps (2 Sam. 12:20, 14:2).

11. One was prohibited from shaving one's hair or beard or cutting one's body. These were condemned as heathen (Lev. 19:27-28, 21:5; Deut. 14:1; Job 1:20; Isa. 22:12; Jer. 16:6, 41:5, 47:5, 48:37; Ezek. 7:18; Amos 8:10).
12. One would fast for seven days (Gen. 50:10; 1 Sam. 31:13; 2 Sam. 1:12, 3:35, 12:20-21).
13. Food was provided for the nearest surviving kin since uncleanness from the corpse prevented food from being prepared in the house (Jer. 16:7; Ezek. 24:17, 22; Hos. 9:4). But offering food to the dead was prohibited (Deut. 26:13-14).
14. Funeral lamentations expressed the qualities of the dead person and the magnitude of the survivors' loss and did not focus primarily on religious concepts. These lamentations were offered by the family (Gen. 23:2, 50:10; 2 Sam. 11:26, 19:1,5; 1 Kings 13:30; Jer. 6:26; Amos 5:16, 8:10; Mic. 1:8; Zech. 12:10-14), by subjects (Jer. 22:18,34), by friends (1 Sam. 25:1, 28:3; 2 Sam. 1:11-12, 3:31), by professional poets (2 Sam. 1:17,19-27, 3:33-34; 2 Chron. 35:25; Jer. 9:16f.; Ezek. 32:16; Amos 5:16, 8:10), and by prophets (Jer. 9:9-11,16-21; Ezek. 19:1-14, 26:17-18, 27:2-9,25-36; 28:12-19, 32:2-8; Amos 5:1-2).
15. Mourning was done at graveside (2 Sam. 3:32).

C. The disposition of the body followed certain established patterns.

1. The body was normally buried on the same day that the death occurred (Deut. 21:22-23).
2. The only exception to same-day burial occured with a royal Egyptian cultural funeral and entombment (Gen. 50:2-3,26).
3. Cremation was not practiced as the norm. The only exception was the cremation of Saul and his sons (1 Sam. 31:12; compare 1 Chron. 10:12).
4. Burning of a body was normally reserved for notorious criminals as a punishment (Gen. 38:24; Lev. 20:14, 21:9; Amos 2:1).
5. Incense or perfumes were sometimes burned near the body (2 Chron. 16:14, 21:19; Jer. 3:5).
6. The conditions of burial varied with the wealth and status of the individual (1 Kings 2:10, 11:43, 14:31; 2 Kings 16:20, 23:6; 2 Chron. 28:37; Job 3:14; Isa. 22:16; Jer. 26:23).
7. Commemorative pillars were used to mark the tomb (Gen. 35:20; 2 Sam. 18:18).
8. Burial normally occurred outside of city limits in family-owned sites (Gen. 23, 25:9-10, 47:30, 49:29-

32; 50:13; Josh. 24:30,32; Judg. 8:32, 16:31; 1 Sam. 25:1; 2 Sam. 2:32, 17:23, 19:28, 21:12-14; 1 Kings 2:34, 13:21-22).

D. Capital punishment was used as an instrument for promoting social order (Exod. 15:17, 21:12, 22:17-19, 31:14-15; Lev. 20:1-5,9-16,27, 21:9, 24:15-17).

The Beliefs, Attitudes, and Values Associated with Death in Old Testament Thanatology

A. Humans are unitary beings with material and immaterial aspects [living nepes (Gen. 2:7), dead nepes (Lev. 21:11; Num. 6:6); nepes as a surrogate for the personal pronoun (Gen. 35:18; 1 Sam. 18:1, 19:3; 1 Kings 17:17, 19:4; Job 34:14-15; Ps. 104:29, 146:4; Eccles. 3:19-21, 12:7; Isa. 53:12; Lam. 2:12; Jon. 4:8).

B. Physical death originated when God imposed premature death for Adam and Eve as a consequence of disobedience (Gen. 2:7,17,19, 3:19,22).

C. All life (agricultural, animal, human) partakes in a cyclical birth and death process (Lev. 17:3-4; Josh. 23:14; Ps. 104:30; Eccles. 12:7).

D. Mortality is designed for all creatures. Therefore, death in old age is valued whereas premature death is considered a calamity (Gen. 25:8; Prov. 10:21; Eccles. 3:2).

E. God controls the quality of one's life and the timing and nature of one's death (Deut. 30:15-19; 1 Sam. 2:6; Ps. 13:3-4).

F. Even though mortality is universal now, it will one day be reversed (Gen. 3:19; 2 Sam. 14:14; Job 14:7-12; Eccles. 3:2; Isa. 25:6-8, 26:14, 65:17,20, 66:22-24).

G. Each person lives and dies once.

H. The place of the dead (sheol) is variously described as:
   1. a place of darkness (Job 10:21-22; Ps. 143:3)
   2. a place of silence (Ps. 94:17, 115:17)
   3. a place of forgetfulness (Ps. 88:12)
   4. a place of separation from God (Ps. 6:5, 88:3-5, 10-12; Isa. 38:18-19)
   5. a place where one is uninformed about the events that take place among the living on earth (Job 14:21; Eccles. 9:5-6, 10)

6. a place of reunion with kin (Gen. 15:15, 25:8; 2 Sam. 12:23)
7. a place with inhabitants (Job 26:5; Isa. 1:10-11; Ezek. 32:17-32)
8. a place where both the good and evil people go (1 Sam. 28:19; Job 3:17-19; Eccles. 9:5f.; Isa. 14:15; Ezek. 32:23; compare Josephus's Bell. Jud. 3, 8.5)
9. miscellaneous general descriptions (1 Sam. 2:6; 2 Sam. 22:5-6; Job 18:5-21, 22:24, 28:22, 30, 30:23, 33:18, 38:17; Ps. 9:13, 16:10, 18:4-5, 115:17, 143:3; Lam. 3:6)
10. a place of minimal existence but not personal annihilation (Job 26:5-6; Ps. 6:5; Isa. 14:9-10; Jer. 51:39; Ezek. 32:17-32).

I. There is a two-way theology of retribution after death (Job 19:25; Ps. 16:10, 17:15; Prov. 14:32; Eccles. 12:14; Isa. 24:21, 26:14-19, 50:11; Ezek. 37; Dan. 12:2).

J. A future day of universal judgment is coming (Ps. 73:27; Isa. 66:15-16; Ezek. 39:21; Joel 3:1-2; Zeph. 3:8; Zech. 14).

K. There are some positive considerations of death (which allow for an interpretation of a death as being "good"; compare Gen. 15:15, 25:8, 46:30; Num. 23:10; Job 5:26; Isa. 65:17-18,20; Jer. 34:4-5):

1. because death does not negate hope (Job 19:25-27; Ps. 16:9-11, 17:15, 49:12-15; 75:24-26)
2. because one can leave behind a good reputation, posterity, or inheritance (Prov. 10:7; Isa. 56:3-5)
3. because death motivates the wise person to learn (Ps. 90:12-14)
4. because it rescues the sufferer from misery (Num. 11:15, 20:3; 1 Kings 19:4; Job 3:19-26, 7:15; Eccles. 3:2, 4:2-3; Jon. 4:3-8)
5. because God abbreviates the life of a wicked person (Gen. 6:6-7; Num. 32:13-14)
6. because there is community solidarity even after the individual's death (Gen. 12:1-3,7, 13:14-16, 24:1-9, 48:21; Exod. 19:6; Num. 20:1-13; Deut. 3:23-28, 31:2-3; 34:1-8)
7. because one can be remembered by the living after he or she is dead (Ps. 41:5; Prov. 10:7; Isa. 56:3-5)
8. because the Lord controls how and when one dies (Gen. 27:2; Deut. 31:14; 2 Sam. 14:14; 1 Kings 2:1, 19:4; 2 Kings 2:3,5,9; Job 1:21; Eccles. 8:8).

L. There are some negative considerations of death (which allow for an interpretation of a death as being "bad"):

1. if it is premature (1 Sam. 2:31; 2 Sam. 18:32-33; Job 36:13-14; Prov. 10:21, 11:19; Isa. 38:1-3,10,12
2. if it is violent (Gen. 4:10; 1 Sam. 15:32, 28:15-20; 1 Kings 2:28-33; Ezek. 28:8; Amos 7:11)
3. if there is no surviving heir (Gen. 15:2-3; Ruth 4:10; 2 Sam. 28:18; Job 5:25-26; Isa. 53:10)
4. if it is death by suicide (Judg. 9:54, 16:30; 1 Sam. 31:4-5,14; 2 Sam. 1:9, 7:23; 1 Kings 16:18).
5. if it is the death of an infant (2 Sam. 12:14-24; 1 Kings 3:16-28, 14:17-18; 2 Kings 4:1-37; Isa. 65:20)
6. if it is death as divine judgment (Ezek. 32:20-36; Nah. 1:14).

M. Any occultic communication with the dead is expressly forbidden (Exod. 22:18; Lev. 20:27; Deut. 14:1, 18:11, 26:14; 1 Sam. 28:7; Ps. 106:28; Eccles. 9:6; Isa. 16:22, 18:8, 65:4).

N. There are numerous descriptions of death:

1. as blessedness (Ps. 116:15)
2. as departure (Gen. 35:18; Ruth 1:17)
3. as sleep (Job 7:21, 11:18, 20:11; Ps. 13:3; Dan. 12:2)
4. as expiration (Gen. 25:8,17, 35:29, 49:33; Job 14:10, 27:3, 31:39; Ps. 104:29; Jer. 15:9; Lam. 1:19)
5. as spilled water (2 Sam. 14:14)
6. as the harvest of a reaper (Jer. 9:22)
7. as a personified being or power (2 Sam. 22:5-6; Job 18:13; Ps. 18:4-5, 49:14-15; Hab. 2:5).

O. There are chronic, degenerative diseases in life. Some of these diseases are divinely healed but most are not (Exod. 23:26; Lev. 14:2-32; 2 Chron. 21:19; Jer. 16:4).

P. When one is separated from participation in life's activities, he or she experiences an existential quality of deadness (Ps. 6:5, 31:12, 48:14, 68:20; 88, 115:17; Eccles. 9:4-5; Isa. 59:10).

Q. Societies use familiar customs or rites of passage in order to acknowledge the death of a member (Gen. 37:34; Josh. 7:6; 1 Sam. 4:12; 2 Sam. 1:11, 3:31, 12:40, 14:2, 15:30, 19:5; Esther 4:3; Ps. 79:3; Eccles. 6:3; Isa. 14:19-20; Jer. 7:32, 8:1-3, 22:19; Ezek. 24:17,23; Mic. 1:10).

The Customs, Practices, and Experiences Associated
with Death in Intertestamental Thanatology[68]

A. Dead bodies must be buried (Tob. 1:17-19, 2:3-4,7-8,
   3:6, 4:3-4, 12:12-13, 14:2,9,11-14).

B. Dead bodies are ceremonially unclean (Tob. 2:5-9).

C. Mourning among the survivors involved:
   1. wearing sackcloth (2 Macc. 3:19)
   2. putting soil on one's head (2 Macc. 10:25, 14:15)
   3. fasting for seven days (Jth. 8:5-6, 16:24, 38:17)
   4. refraining from using perfumes and soaps (Jth. 10:3)
   5. offering funeral lamentations (1 Macc. 9:21; Tob.
      2:5-6, 10:4,7).

D. The survivors are obliged to commemorate the dead (Tob.
   1:17-19; Sir. 7:33, 22:11-12). This commemoration can be
   done by marking the tomb with monuments (1 Macc.
   13:27-30) and by putting food and drink at the grave
   of the dead person (Bar. 6:26; Sir. 30:18; Tob. 4:17;
   compare Wisdom of Ahiqar) and by praying or sacrificing
   for the dead (2 Macc. 12:38-46).

The Beliefs, Attitudes, and Values Associated
with Death in Intertestamental Thanatology

A. All human beings are mortal (Ecclus. 17:30, 25:24; Jubi-
   lees 3:28).

B. It is the Lord who controls, causes, and times death
   (Tob. 1:17-18,21, 3:6, 4:19, 6:13, 13:2, 14:10-11). The
   Lord is the divine judge (Tob. 3:2, 5:6, 13:10, 14:10;
   3 Macc. 2:3) who uses divine timing (Tob. 1:17-19, 4:19,
   13:2).

C. Sometimes demons can kill human beings (Tob. 3:8, 6:14-
   15, 8:2-3).

D. Historically, death is the result of the devil (Wisd. 1:12-
   13, 2:23-24). Historically, death is the result of the
   woman's disobedience (Ecclus. 25:24). Also, death is the
   historic result of Adam's disobedience (Esdras 3:21).

E. Since death can be viewed as a divine judgment (Tob.
   1:17-18,21, 3:4,8, 6:13-15, 14:10-11), then premature
   death can be viewed as a calamity or great misfortune
   (Tob. 1:8-9,19, 2:8, 3:10, 6:15, 8:14, 10:3). However,

premature death can be avoided by righteous conduct (Tob. 4:9-10, 12:9, 14:10-11; compare Prov. 10:2). If one dies prematurely as a righteous person under persecution, this is a special reward (Wisd. 3:4-5, 4:7-14; Test Abr. 14). If one dies as a martyr, he or she will have no fear of death (Test. Abr. 1:10, 7, 8:30, 9, 14, 16, 18, 19:19f., 20). Physical death is only feared by wicked people (Wisd. 2:1,6,10,21-22, 3:10, 4:20).

F. One can find comfort in death:

    1. if they die in old age (Tob. 6:15)
    2. if they are survived by numerous posterity (Ecclus. 44:1,7-9)
    3. if they are remembered after they are dead (Ecclus. 44:1-2,12-13)
    4. if death brings them relief from misery in life (Tob. 3:6,10,13).
    5. if they die as a heroic martyr witnessing to the faith (2 Macc. 6:23-28)
    6. if they have resisted apostasy (which guarantees future physical resurrection, 2 Macc. 7:10-11,23).

G. When someone is physically, spiritually, or emotionally ill, he or she is approaching death and needs divine healing (Tob. 3:4,16, 5:10, 6:4,7-8, 7:7, 8:16, 11:6, 12:3,9,14, 14:11).

H. If they are disabled by their illness and cannot participate in life's activities, they experience a quality of deadness (Tob. 5:10, 12:6; Sir. 14:16, 22:11, 41:4).

I. Even if one is experiencing severe human anguish, suicide is always a shameful way of coping with suffering (Tob. 3:10).

J. Satan is the arch-cause of all human trouble (Wisd. 2:23-24; Life of Adam and Eve 12-16, IQS III, 17-22; 1 Ethiopian Book of Enoch 54:6; compare 1 Chron. 21:1; 2 Sam. 24:1; Job 1-2).

K. When one of the faithful does die, the faithful survivors are obliged to treat the corpse with honor and ceremony (Tob. 2:6, 4:2-3,17, 12:12-13, 14:2,9,11-12); but they are not allowed to engage in any cult of the dead (Tob. 4:7; Sir. 30:18; Bar. 6:26).

L. The place of the dead is described as hades or sheol (Tob. 3:10, 4:19, 13:2):

1. a place of darkness (Tob. 4:10, 5:10, 14:10; 1 Enoch 46:6)
2. an eternal place (Tob. 3:6, 14:10)
3. a subterranean place (Tob. 3:6,10, 4:19, 6:15, 13:2, 14:10; Wisd. 16:13)
4. a place of inactivity (Tob. 5:10, 12:6; Sir. 14:16, 22:11, 41:4)
5. a place of destruction and poverty (Tob. 8:21, 13:2, 14:10; Sir. 33:20-24)
6. a snare to the living (Tob. 14:10).

M. The truly righteous experience an existential form of eternal life before they die which continues on after death (1 QH III, 10-22; IV, 5, 7, 16-17, 29-31; VI, 29-34; VII, 22-23; X, 3-4; XI, 3, 10-13; XIV, 24; XV, 17; XVII, 15; IQSb IV, 12-14; V, 23).

N. The righteous who have been oppressed or persecuted are vindicated, exalted, rewarded, and resurrected after death while the wicked are judged and punished (a severe two-way theology) for their character and deeds in life (Ass. Moses 9-10; Test. Jud. 25; Wisd. 2:4-5, 3:1, 4:7-9, 5:15; Susanna; Sim. Enoch; 1 Macc. 2:1-28,49-68, 6; 2 Macc. 7, 9; 2 Bar. 49-51; 1 Enoch 22:94-104,108; 3 Macc.; Psalms of Sol.; 4 Ezra 7; Sib. Or. 4; Test. Benj. 10; Qumran Hymn Scroll 2:20-30,31-37, 3:19-23, 4:5-5:4, 5:20-6:24, 7:6-25, 11:3-14; IQS 3.13-4.26; Mandate of Hermas; Test. Asher; 2 Baruch 50:2; Jos. Antiq. XVIII, 14; Bell. Jud. II, 154-163; III, 374; CDS 2, I.20; 2, II.6f.; 3, I.20; IQS 10, I.18; 11, II.7-9; IQH 13, II.17f.; IQM 15, II.1f.; 1QH 8, II.4f).

O. There is an intermediate state after death before resurrection (4 Ezra 7:32,75-101; 2 Bar. 21:23, 30:2). This state is a purgatorial phase (1 Enoch 22:9-13). After death there is a two-way retribution (2 Esd. 7:6,72,102-105; Josephus Wars II, 8.14; Antiq. XVIII, 1.3; also compare Enoch, Sib. Or., Apoc. Peter, Apoc. Paul, Test. Abr.).

P. In the consummation of the world, apostate Israel will experience future conversion (Tob. 13:5-6,10,13,15, 14:5,7). At this time, gentile nations will make a pilgrimage to Jerusalem (Tob. 13:13, 14:6; Enoch 90:28-33; Sib. Or. 3.703-31). Jerusalem will then become the center of cosmic-divine activity (Tob. 1:4, 13:10; Wisd. 9:8; Sib. Or. 3.663, 3.772; Jub. 23:22; 1 Enoch 26:4). Jerusalem will become the site of an eternal temple (Tob. 14:5; 1 Enoch 90:27-29; Test. Benj. 9:2; 2 Bar. 4:2-4; Sib. Or. 3.98-104, 5.414-33; Jub. 1:17). This temple will be set in a bejeweled city (Tob. 13:16-18, 14:5).

The Practices, Customs, and Experiences Associated with Death in New Testament Thanatology

A. After someone died, extensive preparations were made to the body (Matt. 27:59; Luke 23:56; John 11:44, 19:39-40).

B. The body was usually unembalmed and carried on a bier (Luke 7:14; Acts 5:10).

C. When someone died, angels were present at their death (Luke 16:22).

D. The way in which the corpse was treated did not help or hinder the deceased person (Matt. 8:22).

E. The body would be buried (Matt. 8:21, 14:12; Luke 9:59-60; Acts 5:6,9-10; 1 Cor. 15:4) and then physical decomposition would set in (John 11:39).

The Attitudes, Values and Beliefs Associated with Death in New Testament Thanatology

A. Human death is historically the result of Adam's disobedience (Rom. 5:19,21, 6:22-23, 8:19-22; 1 Cor. 15:22).

B. Human death may be self-inflicted (Matt. 27:3-10), may be invited by disobedient living (1 Cor. 11:30; 1 John 5:16-17), or may result from capital punishment (Matt. 20:18).

C. When a person becomes ill, God does not always choose to heal them (2 Cor. 12:7-19). However, pain interventions are an alternative to complete suffering (John 19:29).

D. On occasion, a person may experience a near-death or out-of-body experience (Acts 8:39-40; 2 Cor. 5:8, 12:2-4; Phil. 2:27-30; Rev. 1:10).

E. Although death can be described as a personified power (Rom. 5:4, 6:9; 1 Cor. 15:26; Heb. 2:14; Rev. 6:8, 20:14) and its fear can be manipulated by Satan (Heb. 2:14-15), Christ has vanquished the ultimate power of death (John 11:26; 1 Cor. 15:25-26, 53-55).

F. Death has various descriptions in the New Testament:

    1. blessedness (Phil. 1:21; 2 Cor. 5:8)
    2. sleep (John 11:11-14; 1 Thess. 4:13)
    3. relief (Rev. 9:6)
    4. departure (Phil. 1:23; 2 Tim. 4:6)

      5. transfer from a bodily house to a heavenly dwelling (2 Cor. 5:1)

      6. ultimate separation from God (Rev. 20:6,14).

G. The place of the dead is frequently described (Matt. 25:31-46; Luke 16:19,31; John 14:1-3; 2 Cor. 5:1-2), often with eternal qualities (Rom. 6:23; 1 Tim. 1:10; Rev. 20:14).

H. Two radically distinct existential identities are offered in this life whereby belief in Christ results in spiritual/eternal life and unbelief in Him results in spiritual/eternal death (Matt. 25:31-47; John 1:4, 3:36, 5:24, 8:21,51-53, 10:17-18, 11:25-26, 12:23-24; Rom. 7:10,24, 8:6; 1 John 3:14-16).

I. Every person is destined to experience eternal blessing or eternal torment (Matt. 5:22,29-30, 7:9,19-23, 8:12, 10:28, 11:22-24, 12:31-32, 13:40-42, 22:13; Mark 3:29, 9:43-48; Luke 16:19-31; John 14:2-3; 2 Thess. 1:6-9; 2 Pet. 2:4-21; Jude 6-7,13-15; Rev. 7:17).

J. Jesus Christ is going to return to the human sphere again (Matt. 13:26, 24:42-44, 26:64; Luke 12:39-40; 1 Thess. 5:2; Jude 14-15; Rev. 19:11-16).

K. Physical death is going to end one day as an active principle in human experience (Rev. 20:10,14; 21:3-4).

L. There will be a resurrection to life (Luke 14:13-14; John 5:28-29; Phil. 3:10-14; Heb. 11:35; Rev. 20:6) and a resurrection to damnation (Matt. 7:13-14, 25:46; John 3:18, 5:29, 8:24; Rev. 20:5,11-13). The premillennial program of resurrections is (1 Cor. 15:20-24):

    1. Jesus Christ's historic resurrection

    2. the church's translation at the rapture (1 Thess. 4:16)

    3. resurrection of tribulation saints and Old Testament saints at the second advent prior to the millennium (Isa. 26:19; Dan. 12:2; Rev. 20:3-5)

    4. the final resurrection of the wicked (Rev. 20:5,11-14).

The first three phases of this program are the resurrection to life (the first resurrection) whereas the last phase is the resurrection to damnation (the final resurrection).

M. God alone is immortal (1 Tim. 6:16).

N. Humans live once and die once (John 8:58; Heb. 7:3, 9:27).

INSTRUCTIONAL MATERIALS

Although the field of thanatology is quite young, there are nonetheless some excellent materials that can facilitate the biblical death-education process. Major recommendations for books, articles, and audiovisuals dealing with death are given in the attached bibliography. Selections from the bibliography can be used by a church to create a reference, training, and distribution center. These materials should include training resources for the spiritual care-giving team as well as brief distributive and listening guides for families.

PERSONNEL

Who will comprise the team of spiritual care-givers to carry out the ministry of biblical death education through the church? Pastors should be primary candidates as active team members. The pastors should at least help train volunteers and consult on special cases. Lay educational leaders, elders, deacons, and deaconesses should be challenged for involvement. If these lay leaders are not available for active participation with dying and bereaved parishioners, they should at least take training for the periodic cases in which they must be involved. The core of personnel will come from volunteers who feel burdened for this work.

Whenever parishioners suffer acute loss and work through their grief well, they should be challenged to share their insight and experience (2 Cor. 1:3-4). They may be able to articulate their reactions and adjustments to a counseling group, a training seminar for volunteers, or an individual who is experiencing acute grief. These parishioners who have personally suffered loss and who have been helped by caring people are potential recruits for ministry to the aged, dying, and bereaved.

It would be best if someone on the team functioned as the team coordinator. This person should be experienced in death education and bereavement counseling. This person could be a minister, nurse, social worker, physician, or competent nonprofessional.

EDUCATIONAL SETTING

Where does death education take place? It can take place wherever and whenever people express interest and need for such ministry. Sermons and devotionals can address major thanatological subjects. Lessons in the educational classroom can focus on death, loss, and grief. Seminars can handle this topic on a weekend, weekly, or monthly format. These seminars could be for church leaders or parents. It is especially important that the church help parents explain death to their children at home so that children have a wholesome view of sickness, grief, and death. Death education and bereavement counseling may take place in a clinical setting. When visiting a parishioner in the hospital, the care-giver should be especially sensitive to roommates and fellow patients who want to be included in their ministry.

"THE FLOWER FADETH"

This curriculum design presents theoretical concepts about biblical death education for the church. The theories have led to practice in pastoral, educational, hospice, and counseling ministries. The theory and practice of this ministry has suggested the need for an actual curriculum to be used in the church. As a result, a pastoral-care curriculum for biblical death education in the church has been created. The project has pursued a basically descriptive survey methodology. It has sought to observe, correlate, and integrate positively the contemporary thanatology practice of death education with substantive biblical theology and pastoral ministry.

The objective for the whole curriculum is to facilitate a holistic pastoral and biblical death-education program in the local church. This objective was designed to be accomplished through audio, visual, and written materials accompanied by personal instruction and ministry experiences. The intermediate objectives are to develop a synoptic view of biblical thanatology, to interact with age-appropriate themes of biblical thanatology, and to develop the leadership skills for effective involvement in church-related ministries to the aging, dying, and bereaved.

An overview of curriculum components illustrates the nature of the teaching resources. Further detail is included in the individual resources of the curriculum.

CONCLUSION

The modern church holds a strategic advantage for nurturing the aging, dying, and bereaved person in our society. The caring church can embrace the best of thanatological research and integrate it with sound religious belief and ministry. Through a holistic program of biblical death education in the church, the lay religious community can be mobilized to extend

the scope of pastoral care. In order to improve the quality
of spiritual care for the aging, dying, and bereaved, the
evangelical church should consider several recommendations:
(1) offer clergy training opportunities in pastoral gerontol-
ogy/thanatology; (2) produce Christian education resources
relevant to thanatology; and (3) sponsor church-based hospice teams. By this special form of caring, a fresh dimension
of divine love can become evident to humans in need.

NOTES

1. The Foundation of Thanatology (630 W. 168th St.,
New York NY 10032). The Center for Death Education and
Research (University of Minnesota, 1167 Social Science Build-
ing, Minneapolis MN 55455). Laboratory for the Study of Life-
Threatening Behavior (University of California at Los Angeles,
School of Medicine). Center for Studies of Suicide Prevention
(National Institute of Mental Health). Omega Journal of Death
and Dying (Baywood Publishing Co., 120 Marine St., Farm-
ingdale NY 11735). Thanatology Today, professional newslet-
ter (Atcom Building, 2315 Broadway, New York NY 10024).
Advances in Thanatology, successor to Journal of Thanatology
(Foundation of Thanatology, 630 W. 168th St., New York NY
10032). Archives of the Foundation of Thanatology (Foundation of Thanatology, 630 W. 168th St., New York NY 10032).
Robert J. Fulton, A Bibliography of Death, Grief, and Bereavement I, II (Center for Death Education and Research,
University of Minnesota, 1167 Social Science Building, Minne-
apolis MN 55455). L.L. Sell, Death & Dying: An Annotated
Bibliography (Tiresias Press, 116 Pinehurst Ave., New York
NY 10033). National Hospice Organization (1311A Dolley Madison Blvd., McLean VA 22101). Simple Death and Burial Soci-
eties; see Manual of Death Education and Simple Burial and
A Directory of Funeral and Memorial Societies (Burnsville,
S.C.: Celo Press, 1977).

2. There are various examples of individual patient
concerns. One example would be physiological concerns such
as the psychosomatic aspects of disease pathology. See S.C.
Kobassa and M.C. Puccetti, "Personality and Social Resources
in Stress Resistance," Journal of Personality and Social Psychology 45:4 (1983), 839-850. Another example would be psychosocial concerns such as family adjustments to loss. See
R.S. Miller and H.M. Lefcourt, "Social Intimacy: An Important
Moderator of Stressful Life Events," American Journal of Community Psychology 11:2 (1983), 127-139. A final example
would be theological concerns such as beliefs in the afterlife.
See J.A. Arlow, "Scientific Cosmogony, Mythology, and Immortality," Psychoanalytic Quarterly 51:2 (1982), 177-195.

3. There are various examples of theoretical issues. One example would be legal issues such as the definition of "clinical death." M.R. Goodman and M.H. Aung, "Cerebral Death: Theological, Judicial, and Medical Aspects." Heart and Lung 315 (May-June 1978), 329-338. Another example would be ethical issues such as self-termination and the heroic use of life-support equipment. N.J. Osgood, "Suicide in the Elderly: Are We Heeding the Warnings?" Postgraduate Medicine 72:2 (1982), 123-130. Another example would be parapsychological issues such as the psychodynamics of near-death and out-of body experiences. B. Greyson, "The Psychodynamics of Near-Death Experiences," The Journal of Nervous and Mental Disease 171:6 (1983), 376-381. A final example would be cultural issues such as the development and function of rites de passage in societies. E.M. Zuesse, "The Absurdity of Ritual," Psychiatry 46 (February 1983), 40-50.

4. There are various examples of interventional techniques. One example would be palliative pharmacology (such as the use of Brompton's mixture, heroin, or morphine drugs). Another example would be counseling (such as the identification of grief stages).

5. There are various examples of institutional modifications. One example would be altering the traditional curriculum of medical/nursing schools. J. Robbins, "Careers-Care of the Dying: A Universal State," Nursing Mirror 154 (March 1982), 52. S. Caty, B. Downe-Wamboldt, and D. Tamlyn, "Attitudes to Death: Implications for Education," Dimensions in Health Service 59:8 (1982), 20-21; I.E. Thompson, C.P. Lowther, D. Doyle, et al., "Learning About Death: A Project Report from the Edinburgh University Medical School," Journal of Medical Ethics 7:2 (1981), 62-66. Another example would be administering liaison between traditional hospitals/nursing homes and alternative health-care facilities such as hospices. A. Bowling, "The Hospitalisation of Death: Should More People Die At Home?" Journal of Medical Ethics 9:3 (1983), 158-161; M.E. Lauer, R.K. Mulhern, J.M. Wallskog, B.M. Camitta, "A Comparison Study of Parental Adaptation Following a Child's Death at Home or in the Hospital," Pediatrics 71:1 (1983), 107-112; R.K. Mulhern, M.E. Lauer, R.G. Hoffman, "Death of a Child at Home or in the Hospital: Subsequent Psychological Adjustment of the Family," Pediatrics 71:5 (1983), 743-747; A. Munley, C.S. Powers, J.B. Williamson, "Humanizing Nursing Home Environments: The Relevance of Hospice Principles," International Journal of Aging and Human Development 15:4 (1982), 263-284; J.M. Whitfield, R.E. Siegel, A.D. Glicken, R.J. Harmon, L.K. Powers, E.J. Goldson, "The Application of Hospice Concepts to Neonatal Care," American Journal of Diseases of Children 136:5 (1982), 421-424; L.M. Mathew, D.W. Jahnigen, J.R.

Scully, P. Rempel, T.J. Meyer, F.M. LaForce, "Attitudes of House Officers Toward a Hospice on a Medical Service," Journal of Medical Education 58:10 (1983), 772-777; J.R. Machek, "Hospice: New Opportunities for Ministry," Bulletin of the American Protestant Hospital Association 43:2 (1979), 63-67. Another example would be offering social services and insurance coverage to people who choose to die at home. A final example would be engaging churches and synagogues in death education and group counseling.

6. The text of First Thessalonians, fifth chapter (23-24), is significant to the concept of holism. The text reads: "And the very God of Peace sanctify you wholly; and I pray your whole spirit and soul and body be preserved blameless unto the coming of our Lord Jesus Christ. Faithful is He that calleth you, who also will do it" (AV). The text refers to wholeness twice as well as identifying all three major dimensions of the human being. Further, the reference to the God of Peace is no doubt that familiar Hebraic idiom that pictures God as the God of wellness, wholeness, completeness, and peaceful togetherness. Since God Himself is a perfectly balanced and truly integrated being, it is no surprise that He yearns for our restoration and preservation in wholeness. His desire that we be morally yielded to Him, or sanctified, pertains to every level of our being. He will be faithful to His stated agenda to bring us to holy wholeness in the presence of Christ.

7. Right living before God is seen as militating against premature death (Exod. 20:12; Ps. 103:14; Hos. 13:14; Prov. 10:2; Hab. 1:12; Jon. 2:6; Tob. 1:22, 4:9-11, 8:7, 16-17, 12:9, 13:2, 14:10; Heb. 5:7). Conversely, wrong living is seen as inviting premature death (Num. 16:29-30; Job 36:14; Eccles. 7:17; 1 Cor. 11:30; 1 John 5:16-17).

8. Earlier than Old English culture, the Greeks saw a similar holism. It was Hippocrates who prefaced his medical oath to the gods. It was Plato who insisted that one must treat the mind and body of a sick person for effective healing.

9. Luke, the only physician known in biblical literature, followed our Lord's spiritual holism. Among the synoptic writers, Luke's gospel includes fewer references to physical healing than any other. His message may be a model for medical care--the needs of the physical body are not to be seen as superseding the needs of the whole person.

10. J. Epperly, "The Cell and the Celestial: Spiritual Needs of Cancer Patients," Journal of the Medical Association of Georgia 72:5 (1983), 374.

11. Ibid., 375.

12. J.G. Zimring, "When Is the Physician 'Playing God'?" Journal of the American Geriatric Society 28:9 (1980), 419-421.

13. M.W. Lusk, "The Psychosocial Evaluation of the Hospice Patient," Health and Social Work 8:3 (1983), 210-218.

14. "We must be much more concerned about training health professionals in interpersonal skills, such as education, counseling, and relaxation techniques. This is especially true for those fields in which the primary emphasis has been on the acquisition of biomedical information and technical skills . . . they [physicians] must be able to educate and counsel patients about the medical interventions and technical procedures which they perform . . . the provision of education and brief psychotherapies [to patients] tended to reduce cost, while also reducing morbidity and mortality." J. Westermeyer, "Education and Counseling in Hospital Care," American Journal of Public Health 72:2, 127-128. These recommendations for improving physicians' training closely parallel necessary changes for clergy training.

15. J.A. Shelly, "Spiritual Care: Planting Seeds of Hope," Critical Care Update 9:12 (1982), 7-17.

16. J.M. Liaschenko, "Assessment of Anxiety and Depression in the Dying Patient," Topics in Clinical Nursing 2:4 (1981), 39-45.

17. M.W. Lusk, "The Psychosocial Evaluation of the Hospice Patient," Health and Social Work 8:3 (1983), 210-218.

18. L. Ock-Ja, "A Study on Deathbed and Death--Comparison of Clergyman with Medical Man," Taehan Kanho/Korean Nurse 21:2 (1982), 76-78.

19. J.P. Geyman, "Dying and Death of a Family Member," Journal of Family Practice 17:1 (1983), 125-134.

20. E.M. Lamb, "Christian Principles in the Care of the Dying," Australian Nurses Journal 11:7 (1982), 3.

21. N.E. Carson, "How to Succeed in Practice by Really Trying--Guidelines for the Care of Dying Patients," Australian Family Physician 12:2, 124-125.

22. P.B. Friel, "Death and Dying," Annals of Internal Medicine 97:5 (1982), 767-71.

23. Palliative care emphasizes the management of pain and disease symptoms. Curative care emphasizes the unceasing attempt to remove the disease. The former model will utilize a wide range of drug therapies and holistic interventions even if it may invite the patient's death a week or two earlier than traditional curative medicine. The latter model will utilize a more conservative range of drug therapies, will focus on physiological pathologies, and will propose surgery, radiation, or artificial life support in resistance to the disease. In sum, palliative care places the priority on the quality of life while curative care puts it on quantity of life. C.M. Parkes, "Terminal Care: Evaluation of Effects in Surviving Family of Care Before and After Bereavement," Postgraduate Medical Journal 59 (February 1983), 73-78.

24. The greatest spiritual "cure" in Christianity is genuine eternal redemption in Jesus Christ. While this is the foundation of evangelical ministry, it cannot be the sole criterion for the spiritual care of the dying person. For instance, many dying people have already been converted to Christ when they receive their terminal diagnosis. This does not justify spiritual care-providers ignoring the dying person simply because they are already "right with God." On the contrary, there may be many spiritual needs beyond conversion for this dying person--confirming the faith; challenging doubts; borrowing security from familiar songs, sacraments, Scripture, and heritage; doing unfinished business, and coping with guilt; reconciling relationships; family counseling; networking to meet the needs of the grieving family; and answering the questions of helplessness, worthlessness, and social isolation. For those who come to be converted to Christ during their illness, there is a full range of discipleship, nurture, and edification ministries suitable to them. Even for those who never believe, there is a need to clarify the alternatives and guide toward spiritual decisions. Ministries to the unbelieving will often lead to ministries with the family, to volunteers, and to the medical team.

25. S.K. Baum, "Older People's Anxiety About Afterlife," Psychological Reports 52:3 (1983), 895-898.

26. B.H. Glover, "Psychological Needs of the Elderly," Comprehensive Therapy 5:3 (1979), 62-67.

27. J.F. Sanders. T.E. Poole, W.T. Rivero, "Death Anxiety Among the Elderly," Psychological Reports 46:1 (1980), 53-54.

28. C.E. Eisdorfer and W. Keckich, "The Normal Psychopathology of Aging," Proceedings of the Annual Meeting

of the American Psychopathological Association 69 (1980), 1-
18.

29. P.R. Wahl, "Therapeutic Relationships with the
Elderly," Journal of Gerontological Nursing 6:5 (1980), 260-
266.

30. D.C. Kennie, "Good Health Care for the Aged,"
Journal of the American Medical Association 249:6 (1983), 770-
773.

31. D.A. Bille, "Educational Strategies for Teaching
the Elderly Patient," Nursing Health Care 1:5 (1980), 256-263.

32. N.J. Osgood, "Suicide in the Elderly: Are We Heeding the Warnings?" Postgraduate Medicine 72:2 (1982), 123-
130.

33. B.A. Devine, "Attitudes of the Elderly toward
Religion," Journal of Gerontological Nursing 6:1 (1980), 679-
687.

34. There are several possible reasons for the sluggish
response of religious care-givers to those who are very ill.
(1) Some care-givers lack a theological foundation for understanding terminal illness and death. Charismatic/Pentacostal
believers and Christian Science practitioners too readily offer
the unrealistic prospect of a miraculous recovery. When such
a reversal does not take place, the dying person can be led
to believe that personal sin or lack of sufficient faith has prevented the healing. Such religious intervention usually causes
more harm than good. (2) Some care-givers lack a priority in
ministry to those who are chronically ill or acutely aged. Our
society has placed such a priority on physical strength and
beauty that the elderly or disabled are often considered less
valuable persons. When this attitude infiltrates a church, it
can create an overcommitment to programs for adolescents,
young adults, and early-career people at the exclusion of
those who are sick or aged. The church that devotes itself
to young, healthy, working parishioners may derive certain
benefits (such as enthusiasm, high energy level for work in
the church, mobility to attend all of the meetings, financial
contributions, and the potential for long-range involvement).
However, God has not called us to make only selective invest-
ments of ourselves in those people who would appear to offer
the highest rate of return. He has called us to nurture all of
His children. (3) Some caregivers lack a priority in ministry
on social compassion in general. In religious groups where
there is an overemphasis on sectarian beliefs and practices,
the basic needs of fellow human beings can be ignored. Jesus

spoke to this point when he told the parable of the Good Sa-
maritan (Luke 10:30-37). He condemned the Jewish clergy for
avoiding the acute needs of the man who was beaten and left
to die along the road. By way of contrast, the common Samar-
itan traveler (who would have been despised by the Jewish
clergy) did stop and tenderly cared for the wounded man.
The Judeo-Christian ethic has always stressed the obligation
to attend the needs of personae miserabile (persons in piti-
able circumstances, widows, orphans, travelers, foreigners;
Deut. 14:29; Mark 12:31; James 1:27; 1 John 3:14-18). The
greater the need is, the greater our obligation becomes. (4)
Some care-givers lack skillful preparation in issues related
to death and dying. Most care-givers have attended or parti-
cipated in many funerals. This is a basic part of life. However, many of these same care-givers have never had significant dialogue with dying people. Perhaps they have rarely
dealt with a person's grief reactions to the loss of an organ,
limb, sensory function, or sexual function as an analogy to
death. The care-giver may be uncomfortable in ministering to
a child who has a fatal illness or who has lost both parents
to death. A care-giver could be unfamiliar with the final
stages of cancer or with the physiology and management of
pain. If he or she has not given ministry priority to the bereaved, he or she may not understand guilt reactions, the
role of anger, psychotic illusions of voices or appearances,
identifications with the deceased, increased morbidity, or
anniversary reactions, etc. If a care-giver is unaware of
his feelings toward his own mortality, then the acute
needs of the dying or bereaved person can be quite unset-
tling. When this is true, the care-giver's frequent longer
visit, with open communication, physical touch, and shared
grief is replaced by the infrequent, perfunctory, lightning-
quick visit, with religious clichés or by phone calls. (5) Some
care-givers lack the time and energy to care adequately for
the aged, dying, and bereaved. It would be ideal for care-
givers to spend two or three open visits a week with those
who are in great need. These visits may last anywhere from
15 minutes to several hours, depending on the cues from the
sick person. Such open visiting could take on the nature of
a friendly conversation, a miniature religious service, or even
an intense counseling session. In any case, regular visiting
from the religious care-giver with this kind of an open agenda would familiarize the care-giver with the actual physical,
emotional, and spiritual state of affairs with the person. Honest communication could take place instead of religious fa-
cades by the spiritual care-provider or the person in need.
Such visiting would also allow the primary care-taker in a
home to leave the sick patient attended in order to do something of interest or necessity. Beyond these times of personal
companionship, the spiritual care-giver should be available by

phone at most times. It is needless to say that this level of
spiritual care involvement is highly supportive. However, it
also becomes apparent that few care-givers can afford the
time and emotional energy it would take to serve numerous
people in this kind of arrangement over several months. While
the initial four causes for substandard spiritual care could
be addressed in theological training institutions or ministerial
associations, the final one must be addressed with the congregational laity in mind. Since it is impossible for any minister to do the work of the church himself, he must concentrate on equipping the people so that they can do the work
of this ministry along with him (Eph. 4:11-13).

35. M.E. O'Brien, "An Identification of the Needs of
Family Members of Terminally Ill Patients in a Hospital Setting," Military Medicine 148 (September 1983), 712-716.

36. E.M. Zuesse, "The Absurdity of Ritual," Psychiatry
4 (February 1983), 40-50.

37. R. Lapwood, "Chaplain to Casualty," British Medical Journal 285 (July 1982), 194-195.

38. R. Dayringer, "The Religious Professionals' Contribution to Health Care," Surgery Annual 15 (1983), 113.

39. Rev. Carl Nighswonger, chaplain in the Chicago-
area hospitals, invited Dr. Elisabeth Kübler-Ross to begin the
research which resulted in her first pioneering book, On
Death and Dying (New York: Macmillan, 1969).

40. Anonymous, "Cabrini Medical Center, New York
City--Terminally Ill Pastoral Care Director Founds Hospice,"
Hospital Progress 61:10 (1980), 28.

41. R. Dayringer, op. cit.

42. R. Winton, "The Role of the Hospital Chaplain,"
The Medical Journal of Australia 1:13 (1982), 540.

43. G.G. Merrill, "Religious Values in Treatment,"
Maryland State Medical Journal 31:12 (1982), 33-34.

44. M. Kelsey, Afterlife: The Other Side of Dying
(New York: Paulist Press, 1979), p. 219.

45. Most churches have a group of people who, because of their unique abilities and interests, carry on the
bulk of the music ministry. Another group bears the main
burden of personal evangelism. Others devote themselves to

the financial and business concerns of the church. Those who are gifted to teach do so with eagerness. Likewise, developing a network of specialized lay care-givers for the aged, dying, and bereaved permits the church to edify itself in love.

46. P. Bermensolo and S. Groenwald, "Are We Death and Dying Our Patients to Death?" Oncology Nursing Forum 5:4 (1978), 8-10; J.W. Worden and A.D. Weisman, "Do Cancer Patients Really Want Counseling?" General Hospital Psychiatry 2:2 (1980), 100-103.

47. L. Videka-Sherman, "Coping with the Death of a Child: A Study Over Time," American Journal of Orthopsychiatry 52:4 (1982), 688-98.

48. C.S. Aneschensel and J.D. Stone, "Stress and Depression: A Test of the Buffering Model of Social Support," Archives of General Psychiatry 39:12 (1982), 1392-1396.

49. J.A. Kotarba even argues that people suffering with chronic pain or terminal illness should find a religious commitment or community of faith if they don't already have one. Kotarba also suggests that health-care providers should help the patients find a religious identity for its medical effect. He advises that pain-care facility administrators should add pastoral counselors to their therapeutic teams. J.A. Kotarba, "Perspections of Death, Belief Systems, and the Process of Coping with Chronic Pain," Social Science and Medicine 17:10 (1983), 681-689.

50. L. Lilliston, P.M. Brown, H.P. Schliebe, "Perceptions of Religious Solutions to Personal Problems of Women," Journal of Clinical Psychology 38:3 (1982), 549-559.

51. A.R. Favazza, "Modern Christian Healing of Mental Illness," American Journal of Psychiatry 139:6 (1982), 728-735; C.R. Sachtleben, "The Role of Belief Systems in Cancer Therapy," Delaware Medical Journal 50:2 (1978), 71-72.

52. As with any new education program in the church, leadership is well advised to proceed thoughtfully with implementation. New programs must always be tailored to individual churches toward their real needs. Leadership must privately clarify its rationale for the new program and its logistical implications. Then formative ideas need to be planted with auxiliary leaders and time given for incubation. When a fair sample of interest has been demonstrated, a gradual program of death education can begin.

53. The health of a family often determines the duration and severity of bereavement. Rather than merely focus

on crisis-intervention strategies, church leaders should seek
to develop healthy families in light of their eventual bereavement experiences. This will allow a family to heal itself more
readily than an expert coming to "fix" them during a bereavement crisis. Developing a team of lay care-giving specialists
is another version of the healthy family healing itself. E. Elizur and M. Kaffman, "Factors Influencing the Severity of
Childhood Bereavement Reactions," American Journal of Orthopsychiatry 53:4 (1983), 668-676. People who are under high
stress suffer less illness when they perceive themselves to be
socially well supported by others. S.C. Kobassa and M.C.
Pucetti, "Personality and Social Resources in Stress Resistance," Journal of Personality and Social Psychology 45:4
(1983), 839-850. Individuals lacking a current intimacy were
found to be prone to higher levels of emotional disturbance
especially when many previous negative or few positive life-
change events had occurred. R.S. Miller and H.M. Lefcourt,
"Social Intimacy: An Important Moderator of Stressful Life
Events," American Journal of Community Psychology 11:2
(1983), 127-139. People must learn to integrate their past
healthy coping adjustments from life-change events with their
new life developments. J.M. Eddy, R.S. St. Pierre, W.F.
Alles, "Life Span Development: Intervention Implications for
Concepts of Aging," Journal of School Health 52:9 (1982),
559-563. Nonpsychiatric people-helpers can and should learn
to do simple stress counseling with people. B.D. Gutnik, "A
Stress Counseling Paradigm for the Nonpsychiatrist," Nebraska Medical Journal 67:3 (1982), 52-54. Family therapy skills
can be very helpful in dealing with terminal illness and death.
M.M. Tousley, "The Use of Family Therapy in Terminal Illness and Death," Journal of Psychosocial Nursing and Mental
Health Services 20:1 (1982), 17-22. People can be somewhat
educated in healthful aging. G.K. Brewer, "Promoting Healthful Aging through Strengthening Family Ties," Topics in Clinical Nursing 3:1 (1981), 45-50.

54. L.E. Lerea and B.F. LiMauro, "Grief Among Health-
care Workers: A Comparative Study," Journal of Gerontology
37:5 (1982), 604-608. J.P. Rafferty, "The Personal Stress of
Working with the Seriously Ill: Impact on the Caregiver,"
Progress in Clinical and Biological Research 121 (1983), 279-
286.

55. A.J. Taylor and A.G. Frazer, "The Stress of Post-
Disaster Body Handling and Victim Identification Work," Jour-
nal of Human Stress 8:4 (1982), 4-12; L.E. Lerea, B.F.
LiMauro, "Grief Among Healthcare Workers: A Comparative
Study," Journal of Gerontology 37:5 (1982), 604-608.

56. J. Roskin, "Coping with Life Changes--A Preventive Social Work Approach," American Journal of Community Psychology 10:3 (1982), 331-340.

57. J.T. Brown, G.A. Stoudemire, "Normal and Pathological Grief," Journal of the American Medical Association 250:3 (1983), 378-382.

58. M.E. Lauer, R.K. Mulhern, J.M. Walskog, B.M. Camitta, "A Comparison Study of Parental Adaptation Following a Child's Death at Home or in the Hospital," Pediatrics 71:1 (1983), 107-112; R.K. Mulhern, M.E. Lauer, and R.G. Hoffman, "Death of a Child at Home or in the Hospital: Subsequent Psychological Adjustment of the Family," Pediatrics 71:5 (1983), 743-747; A. Bowling, "The Hospitalisation of Death: Should More People Die at Home?" Journal of Medical Ethics 9:3 (1983), 158-161.

59. R.E. Clark and E.E. LaBeff, "Death Telling: Managing the Delivery of Bad News," Journal of Health and Social Behavior 23 (December 1982), 366-380; J.L. Anderson, "A Practical Approach to Teaching about Communication with Terminal Cancer Patients," Journal of Medical Education 54:10 (1979), 823-824.

60. S. Berman and S. Villerreal, "Use of a Seminar as an Aid in Helping Interns Care for Dying Children and Their Families," Clinical Pediatrics 22:3 (1983), 175-179.

61. D. Doyle, K.M. Parry, R.G. MacFarlane, "Education in Terminal Care," Journal of the Royal College of General Practitioners 32 (June 1982), 335-338.

62. M.W. Linn, B.S. Linn, and S. Stein. "Impact on Nursing Home Staff of Training About Death and Dying," Journal of the American Medical Association 250:17 (1983), 2332-2335.

63. D.A. Rublee and W.L. Yarber, "Instructional Units of Death Education: The Impact of the Amount of Classroom Time on Changes in Death Attitudes," Journal of School Health 53:7 (1983), 412-415.

64. C. Jacobs, "A Patient Teaching Tool," Cancer Nursing 2:2 (1979), 153-166.

65. D.A. Bille, "Educational Strategies for Teaching the Elderly Patient," Nursing Health Care 1:5 (1980), 256-263.

66. J.A. Hernan, "Effect of a Gerontological Educational Experience on Adolescent Girls' Attitudes toward the Elderly," Journal of Gerontological Nursing 7:1 (1981), 45-49.

67. K. Doherty, S. Stein, and M.W. Linn. "An In-Service Guide for Death Education," Gerontology and Geriatric Education 2:3 (1982), 191-197; J.A. Piemme, "Death Education: A Different Approach," Oncology Nursing Forum 6:1, 4; A.D. Weisman and H.J. Sobel, "Coping With Cancer Through Self-Instruction," Journal of Human Stress 5:1 (1979), 3-8; C.K. Mahan, R.L. Schreiner, and M. Green, "Bibliotherapy: A Tool to Help Parents Mourn their Infant's Death," Health and Social Work 8:2 (1983), 126-132; R.E. Anstett and S.R. Poole, "Bibliotherapy: An Adjunct to Care of Patients with Problems of Living," Journal of Family Practice 17:5 (1983), 845-853.

68. Intertestamental literature such as the Dead Sea Scrolls and Deutero-canonical materials are cited here to complete the historical transition between Old Testament and New Testament literature. There is clearly a superior theological authority in the canonical literature, compared with these intertestamental writings. However, since the intertestamental Jewish community relied heavily on its Old Testament canon, there are significant correlations in thanatological belief.

REFERENCES

The Resources for Biblical Death
Education in the Church

There are numerous excellent resources for death education. Many of these resources are directly or indirectly adaptable for use in a church-based, biblical, death-education program.

Major Reference Sources

The publications below document more than 10,000 resources for the person involved in death education. These resources include books, periodicals, audiovisuals, and public-private helping organizations.

Fecher, V.J. Religion and Aging: An Annotated Bibliography. San Antonio, Tex.: Trinity, 1982.

Fruehling, J.A. Sourcebook on Death and Dying, 1st ed. Chicago: Marquis, 1982.

Fulton, R. Death, Grief, and Bereavement: A Bibliography, vol. 1 (1845-1975), vol. 2 (1975-1980). New York: Arno Press, 1977, 1981.

Peradotto, J. Classical Mythology: An Annotated Bibliographical Survey. Ann Arbor, Mich.: Edwards, 1973.

Sell, I.L. Dying and Death: An Annotated Bibliography. New York: Tiresias, 1977.

Steere, D.T., Jr. The Hospice: A Bibliographical Supplement to NLM Literature Searches. Bethesda, Md.: National Library of Medicine, 1984.

Wass, H., C.A. Corr, R.A. Pacholski, and C.M. Sanders. Death Education: An Annotated Resource Guide. Washington, D.C.: Hemisphere, 1980.

Individual Reference Sources

The publications below document the resources that have been directly supportive of content or concepts in "The Flower Fadeth."

Aguilera, D.C. and J.M. Messick. Crisis Intervention—Theory and Methodology, 4th ed. St. Louis, Mo.: Mosley, 1982.

Anderson, J.K. Life, Death and Beyond. Grand Rapids, Mich.: Zondervan, 1980.

———. "A Practical Approach to Teaching About Communication with Terminal Cancer Patients." Journal of Medical Education 54:10 (1979), 823-824.

Aneschensel, C.S. and J.D. Stone. "Stress and Depression: A Test of the Buffering Model of Social Supports." Archives of General Psychiatry 39:12 (1982), 1392-1396.

Anonymous. "Cabrini Medical Center, New York City—Terminally Ill Pastoral Care Director Founds Hospice." Hospital Progress 61:10 (1980), 28.

Anstett, R.E. and S.R. Poole. "Bibliotherapy: An Adjunct to Care of Patients with Problems of Living." Journal of Family Practice 17:5 (1983), 845-53.

Aries, P. The Hour of Our Death, translated by H. Weaver. New York: Knopf, 1981.

Arlow, J.A. "Scientific Cosmogony, Mythology, and Immortality." Psychoanalytic Quarterly 51:2 (1982), 177-195.

Arteaga, W. Past-Life Visions--A Christian Exploration. New York: Seabury, 1983.

Atchley, R.C. The Social Forces in Later Life. Belmont, Calif.: Wadsworth, 1980.

Bachmann, C.C. Ministering to the Grief Sufferer. Philadelphia: Fortress, 1964.

Bailey, L.R. Biblical Perspectives on Death. Philadelphia: Fortress, 1979.

Bailey, R. Ministering to the Grieving. Grand Rapids, Mich.: Zondervan, 1976.

Bardis, P. History of Thanatology. Washington, D.C.: University Press of America, 1981.

Barnhart, P. Devotions for Patients. Old Tappan, N.J.: Revell, 1983.

Baum, S.K. "Older People's Anxiety About Afterlife," Psychological Reports 5:3 (1983), 895-898.

Bayly, J. "The Christian Attitude to Death." Regent College Cassette no. 203B, Vancouver, B.C., Canada (n.d.).

---. The View from a Hearse. Elgin, Ill.: Cook, 1969.

---. If I Should Die Before I Wake. Elgin, Ill.: Cook, 1976.

---. The Last Thing We Talk About. Elgin, Ill.: Cook, 1979.

Benjamin, A. The Helping Interview, 3rd ed. Boston: Houghton-Mifflin, 1981.

Berman, S. and S. Villarreal. "Use of a Seminar as an Aid in Helping Interns Care for Dying Children." Clinical Pediatrics 22:3 (1983), 175-179.

Bermensolo, P. and S. Groenwald. "Are We Death and Dying Our Patients to Death?" Oncology Nursing Forum 5:4 (1978), 8-10.

Bille, D.A. "Educational Strategies for Teaching the Elderly Patient." Nursing Health Care 1:5 (1980), 256-263.

Bowling, A. "The Hospitalisation of Death: Should More People Die at Home?" Journal of Medical Ethics 9:3 (1983), 158-161.

Bradbury, W. Into the Unknown. Pleasantville, N.Y.: Reader's Digest, 1981.

Brewer, G.K. "Promoting Healthful Aging through Strengthening Family Ties," Topics in Clinical Nursing 3:1 (1981), 45-50.

Brister, C.W. People Who Care. Nashville, Tenn.: Broadman, 1967.

Brooke, T. The Other Side of Death. Wheaton, Ill.: Tyndale, 1979.

Brown, J.T. and G.A. Stoudemire. "Normal and Pathological Grief." Journal of the American Medical Association 250:3 (1983), 378-382.

Bryant, M.D. and C.F. Kemp. The Church and Community Resources. St. Louis, Mo.: Bethany, 1977.

Bryson, H.T. The Reality of Hell and the Goodness of God. Wheaton, Ill.: Tyndale, 1984.

Budge, E.A.W. Osiris and the Egyptian Resurrection. New York: Dover, 1973.

---. The Egyptian Book of the Dead. New York: Dover, 1967.

Buis, H. The Doctrine of Eternal Punishment. Philadelphia: Presbyterian and Reformed, 1957.

Buscalgia, L. The Fall of Freddie the Leaf. Thorofare, N.J.: Slack, 1982.

Campolo, A. The Success Fantasy. Wheaton, Ill.: Victor, 1980.

Caplan, G. Principles of Preventive Psychiatry. New York: Basic Books, 1964.

Carkhuff, R.R. and W.A. Anthony. The Skills of Helping: An Introduction to Counseling. Amherst, Mass.: Human Resource Development, 1976.

Carson, N.E. "How to Succeed in Practice by Really Trying-- Guidelines for the Care of Dying Patients." Australian Family Physician 12:2 (1982), 124-125.

Cassuto, U. Biblical and Oriental Studies. Jerusalem: Magnes, 1975.

---. The Goddess Anath. Jerusalem: Magnes, 1951.

Casteel, J., ed. The Creative Role of Interpersonal Groups in the Church Today. New York: Association, 1968.

Caty, S., B. Downe-Wamboldt, and D. Tamlyn. "Attitudes to Death: Implications for Education," Dimensions in Health Services 59:8 (1982), 20-21.

Chandler, L. Uncle Ike. Nashville, Tenn.: Broadman, 1981.

Chandler, W.M. Trial of Jesus. Atlanta: Harrison, 1908.

Childress, B.F. Priorities in Biomedical Ethics. Philadelphia: Westminster, 1981.

Choron, J. Death and Western Thought. London: Collier Macmillan, 1963.

Clark, R.E. and E.E. LaBeff. "Death Telling: Managing the Delivery of Bad News." Journal of Health and Social Behavior 23 (December 1982), 366-380.

Claypool, J. Tracks of a Fellow Struggler. Waco, Tex.: Word, 1974.

Clements, W.M., ed. Ministry With the Aging. San Francisco: Harper and Row, 1981.

Clinebell, H. Basic Types of Pastoral Counseling. Nashville, Tenn.: Abingdon Press, 1966.

Collins, G. The Rebuilding of Psychology. Wheaton, Ill.: Tyndale, 1977.

Congdon, H.K. The Pursuit of Death. Nashville, Tenn.: Abingdon Press, 1977.

Cotterell, P. What the Bible Teaches about Death. Wheaton, Ill.: Tyndale, 1979.

Cowan, E.L. and L. Gesten. Community Approaches to Intervention. Englewood Cliffs, N.J.: Prentice-Hall, 1978.

Daglish, E.R. Psalm 51 in the Light of Ancient Near Eastern Patternism. Leiden: Brill, 1962.

Davies, N. Human Sacrifice in History and Today. New York: William Morrow, 1981.

Davis, J.J. Paradise to Prison. Grand Rapids, Mich.: Baker, 1975.

Dayle, W.W. "Effects of Supervision in the Training of Non-professional Crisis Intervention Counselors." Journal of Counseling Psychology 24:1 (1977), 72.

Dayringer, R. "The Religious Professionals' Contribution to Health Care." Surgery Annual 15 (1983), 113.

Delitzsch, F. Proverbs, Ecclesiastes, Song of Solomon in Commentary on the Old Testament, vol. 6, edited by C.F. Keil and F. Delitzsch, translated by J. Martin. Grand Rapids, Mich.: Eerdmans, 1872.

Dempsey, D. The Way We Die. New York: McGraw-Hill, 1975.

Detweiler-Zapp, D. and W.C. Dixon. Lay Caregiving. Philadelphia: Fortress, 1982.

Devine, B.A. "Attitudes of the Elderly toward Religion." Journal of Gerontological Nursing 6:11 (1980), 679-687.

Dobihal, E.F., Jr., and C.W. Steward. When a Friend Is Dying. Nashville, Tenn.: Abingdon Press, 1984.

Doherty, K., S. Stein, and M.W. Linn. "An In-Service Guide for Death Education." Gerontology and Geriatric Education 2:3 (1982), 191-197.

Douty, N. The Death of Christ. Swengel, Pa.: Reiner, 1972.

Doyle, D., K.M. Parry, and R.G. MacFarlane. "Education in Terminal Care." Journal of the Royal College of General Practitioners 32 (June 1982), 335-338.

Ebon, M., ed. True Experiences in Communicating with the Dead. New York: Signet, 1968.

Eddy, J.M., R.W. St. Piemme, and W.F. Alles. "Life Span Development: Intervention Implications for Concepts of Aging." Journal of School Health 52:9 (1982), 559-563.

Egan, G. The Skilled Helper. Monterey, Calif.: Brooks-Cole, 1982.

---. Exercises in Helping Skills. Monterey, Calif.: Brooks-Cole, 1982.

Egner, D.C., ed. Morals for Mortals. Grand Rapids, Mich.: Radio Bible Class, 1979.

Eisdorfer, C.E. and W. Keckich. "The Normal Psychopathology of Aging," Proceedings of the Annual Meeting of the American Psychopathological Association 69 (1980), 1-18.

Eliade, M. Death, Afterlife, and Eschatology. New York: Harper, 1967.

Elizur, E. and M. Kaffman. "Factors Influencing the Severity of Childhood Bereavement Reactions." American Journal of Orthopsychiatry 53:4 (1981), 668-76.

Epperly, J. "The Cell and the Celestial: Spiritual Needs of Cancer Patients." Journal of the Medical Association of Georgia 72:5 (1983), 374.

Erikson, E.H. Insight and Responsibility. New York: Norton, 1964.

Ewens, J. and P. Herrington. Hospice. Santa Fe, N.M.: Bear, 1982.

Faber, H. Striking Sails--A Pastoral Psychological View of Growing Older in Our Society, translated by K.R. Mitchell. Nashville, Tenn.: Abingdon Press, 1984.

Faberow, N.L. and E.S. Shneidman, eds. The Cry for Help. New York: McGraw-Hill, 1961.

Favassa, A.R. "Modern Christian Healing of Mental Illness," American Journal of Psychiatry 139:6 (1982), 728-735.

Feifel, H., ed. The Meaning of Death. New York: McGraw-Hill, 1959.

Feinberg, M.R., G. Feinberg, and J.J. Tarrant. Leavetaking. New York: Simon and Schuster, 1978.

Fichter, J. Religion and Pain. New York: Crossroad, 1981.

Frank, J.D. Persuasion and Healing. Baltimore: Johns Hopkins, 1973

Freeman, J.M. Manners and Customs of the Bible. Plainfield, N.J.: Logos, 1972.

Friel, P.B. "Death and Dying," Annals of Internal Medicine 97:5 (1982), 767-771.

Friesen, G. Decision Making and the Will of God. Portland, Ore.: Multnomah, 1980.

Frost, S.E., Jr. The Sacred Writings of the World's Great Religions. New York: McGraw-Hill, 1943.

Fruehling, J.A., ed. Sourcebook on Death and Dying, 1st ed. Chicago: Marquis, 1982.

Garrison, W. Strange Facts About Death. Nashville, Tenn.: Abingdon Press, 1978.

Geary, D.P. How to Deliver Death News. San Francisco, Calif.: Compass, 1982.

Gerstenberger, E.S. and W. Schrage. Suffering, translated by J.E. Steely (Nashville, Tenn.: Abingdon Press, 1977.

Geyman, J.P. "Dying and Death of a Family Member." Journal of Family Practice 17:1 (1983), 125-134.

Gillies, J. A Guide to Caring for and Coping with Aging Parents. Nashville, Tenn.: Nelson, 1981.

Glover, B.H. "Psychological Needs of the Elderly." Comprehensive Therapy 5:3 (1979), 62-67.

Goodman, M.R. and M.H. Aung. "Cerebral Death: Theological, Judicial, and Medical Concepts." Heart and Lung 7:3 (1978), 477-483.

Gray, R.M. and D.O. Moberg. The Church and the Older Person. Grand Rapids, Mich.: Eerdmans, 1962.

Grantham, R.E. Lay Shepherding: A Guide for Visiting the Sick, the Aged, the Troubled, and the Bereaved. Valley Forge, Pa.: Judson, 1980.

Greysons, B. "The Psychodynamics of the Near-Death Experience." Journal of Nervous and Mental Disease 171:6 (1983), 376-378.

Grollman, E. Explaining Death to Children. Boston: Beacon Press, 1967.

---. Talking About Death--A Dialogue Between a Parent and Child. Boston: Beacon Press, 1970.

---. Suicide--Prevention, Intervention, Postvention. Boston: Beacon Press, 1971.

---. Concerning Death: A Practical Guide to the Living. Boston: Beacon Press, 1974.

---. Living When A Loved One Has Died. Boston: Beacon Press, 1977.

---. When Your Loved One Is Dying. Boston: Beacon Press, 1980.

---. What Helped Me When My Loved One Died. Boston: Beacon Press, 1981.

--- and S. Grollman. Caring for Your Aging Parents. Boston: Beacon Press, 1978.

Gordon, C. "Nuzu Tablets," in E.F. Campbell, ed., Biblical Archaeologist Reader, 3rd ed. Garden City, N.Y.: Doubleday, 1970.

Gutnik, B.D. "A Stress Counseling Paradigm for the Nonpsychiatrist." Nebraska Medical Journal 67:3 (1982), 52-54.

Hamilton, M. and H. Reid. A Hospice Handbook. Grand Rapids, Mich.: Eerdmans, 1980.

Hauerwas, S. "Religious Concepts of Brain Death and Associated Problems." Annals of the New York Academy of Sciences 315 (November 1978), 329-338.

Havner, V. Though I Walk Through the Valley. Old Tappan, N.J.: Revell, 1974.

Hellwig, M. What Are They Saying About Death and Christian Hope? New York: Paulist Press, 1978.

Hendricks, R.A. Mythologies of the World. New York: McGraw-Hill, 1973.

Hernan, J.A. "Effect of a Gerontological Educational Experience on Adolescent Girls' Attitudes toward the Elderly." Journal of Gerontological Nursing 7:1 (1981), 45-49.

Hick, J.H. Death and Eternal Life. San Francisco, Calif.: Harper and Row, 1976.

Hill, B. The Near-Death Experience: A Christian Approach. Dubuque, Iowa: Brown, 1981.

Hillers, D. Lamentations in the Anchor Bible, vol. 7A, edited by W.F. Albright and D.N. Freedman. Garden City, N.Y.: Doubleday, 1972.

Holifield, E.B. A History of Pastoral Care in America. Nashville, Tenn.: Abingdon Press, 1983.

Hollway, G.N. E.S.P. and the Superconscious. Louisville, Ky.: Best, 1966.

Humphreys, S.C. and H. King, eds. Mortality and Immortality. New York: Academic Press, 1981.

Irion, P. The Funeral and the Mourners. Nashville, Tenn.: Abingdon Press, 1954.

Jacobs, C. "A Patient Teaching Tool." Cancer Nursing 2:2 (1979), 153-166.

Jungel, E. Death: The Riddle and the Mystery, translated by I. Nicol and U. Nicol. Philadelphia: Westminster, 1974.

Kaiser, O. and E. Lohse. Death and Life, translated by J.E. Steely. Nashville, Tenn.: Abingdon Press, 1979.

Kapleau, P., ed. The Wheel of Death. New York: Harper and Row, 1971.

Kelsey, M. Afterlife--The Other Side of Dying. New York: Paulist Press, 1979.

Kennie, D.C. "Good Health Care for the Aged." Journal of the American Medical Association 249:6 (1983), 770-773.

Kitchen, K. Ancient Orient and the Old Testament. Downers Grove, Ill.: Intervarsity, 1966.

Kobassa, S.C. and M.C. Puccetti. "Personality and Social Resources in Stress Resistance." Journal of Personality and Social Psychology 45:4 (1983), 839-850.

Komroff, M., ed. The History of Herodotus, translated by G. Rawlinson. New York: Tudor, 1939.

Kopp, R. Where Has Grandpa Gone? Grand Rapids, Mich.: Zondervan, 1983.

--. Encounter with Terminal Illness. Grand Rapids, Mich.: Zondervan, 1980.

Kotarba, J.A. "Perceptions of Death, Belief Systems, and the Process of Coping with Chronic Pain." Social Science and Medicine 17:10 (1983), 681-689.

Krieger, D., ed. The Therapeutic Touch: How To Use Your Hands to Help or to Heal. Englewood Cliffs, N.J.: Prestice-Hall, 1979.

Kübler-Ross, E. On Death and Dying. New York: Macmillan, 1969.

---. Letter to a Child with Cancer. Escondido, Calif.: Shanti Nilaya, n.d.

---. "Life, Death, and Life After Death." Shanti Nilaya Cassette no. 1, Escondido, Calif. (n.d.).

Lamb, E.M. "Christian Principles in the Care of the Dying." The Australian Nurses Journal 11:7 (1982), 3.

Landorf, J. "Mourning Song." One Way Cassette Library, Santa Ana, Calif. (1975).

---. Mourning Song. Old Tappan, N.J.: Revell, 1974.

Lapwood, R. "Chaplain to Casualty," British Medical Journal 285 (July 1982), 194-195.

Lauer, M.E., R.K. Mulhern, J.M. Wallskog, and B.A. Camitta. "A Comparison Study of Parental Adaptation Following a Child's Death at Home or in the Hospital." Pediatrics 71:1 (1983), 107-12.

Lerea, L.E. and B.F. LiMauro. "Grief Among Healthcare Workers: A Comparative Study." Journal of Gerontology 37:5 (1982), 604-608.

LeShan, E. Learning to Say Good-By. New York: Avon, 1976.

Levinson, D.J. The Seasons of a Man's Life. New York: Ballantine, 1978.

Lewis, C.S. A Grief Observed. New York: Bantam Books, 1976.

Lewis, J.M. To Be a Therapist. New York: Bruner-Mazel, 1978.

Liaschenko, J.M. "Assessment of Anxiety and Depression in the Dying Patient." Topics in Clinical Nursing 2:4 (1981), 39-45.

Lilliston, L., P.M. Brown, and H.P. Schliebe. "Perceptions of Religious Solutions to Personal Problems of Women." Journal of Clinical Psychology 38:3 (1982), 549.

Linn, M.W., B.S. Linn, and S. Stein. "Impact on Nursing Home Staff of Training About Death and Dying." Journal of the American Medical Association 250:7 (1983), 2332-2335.

Lusk, M.W. "The Psychosocial Evaluation of the Hospice Patient." Health and Social Work 8:3 (1983), 210-218.

Machek, J.R. "Hospice: New Opportunities for Ministry." Bulletin of the American Protestant Hospital Association 43:2 (1979), 63-67.

Mahan, C.K., R.L. Schreiner, and M. Green. "Bibliotherapy: A Tool to Help Parents Mourn Their Infant's Death." Health and Social Work 8:2 (1983), 126-132.

Marshall, C., ed. John Doe, Disciple: Sermons for the Young in Heart. New York: McGraw-Hill, 1963.

Mathew, L.M., D.W. Jahnigen, J.R. Scully, P. Rempel, T.J. Meyer, and F.M. LaForce. "Attitudes of House Officers Toward a Hospice on a Medical Service." Journal of Medical Education 58:10 (1983), 772-777.

McCollum, A.T. The Chronically Ill Child. New Haven, Conn.: Yale University Press, 1981.

McGrath, J.E., ed. Social and Psychological Factors in Stress. New York: Holt, Rinehart, and Winston, 1970.

Mellonie, B. and R. Ingpen. Lifetimes. New York: Bantam Books, 1983.

Merrill, G.G. "Religious Values in Treatment." Maryland State Medical Journal 31:12 (1982), 33-34.

Miller, R.S. and H.M. Lefcourt. "Social Intimacy: An Important Moderator of Stressful Life Events." American Journal of Community Psychology 11:2 (1983), 127-139.

Mills, G. et al. Discussing Death: A Guide to Death Education. Palm Springs, Calif.: ETC, 1982.

Moody, R.A. Life After Life. Harrisburg, Penna.: Stackpole, 1976.

Morgan, E. A Manual of Death Education and Simple Burial. Burnsville, S.C.: Celo, 1977.

Morley, R.A. Death and Afterlife. Minneapolis: Bethany, 1984.

Mulhern, R.K., M.E. Lauer, and R.G. Hoffman. "Death of a Child at Home or in the Hospital: Subsequent Psychological Adjustment of the Family." Pediatrics 71:5 (1983), 743-747.

Munley, A., C.S. Powers, and J.B. Williamson. "Humanizing Nursing Home Environments: The Relevance of Hospice Principles." International Journal on Aging and Human Development 15:4 (1982), 263-284.

Myers, J., ed. Voices From the Edge of Eternity. Old Tappan, N.J.: Spire, 1968.

Neale, R.E. "Explorations in Death Education." Pastoral Psychology 22 (1971), 33-74.

Nickelsburg, G. Resurrection, Immortality, and Eternal Life. Cambridge, Mass.: Harvard University Press, 1972.

Nielsen, N., Jr., et al. Religions of the World. New York: St. Martin's Press, 1983.

Nystrom, C. What Happens When We Die? Chicago: Moody, 1981.

O'Brien, M.E. "An Identification of the Needs of Family Members of Terminally Ill Patients in a Hospital Setting." Military Medicine 148 (September 1983), 712-716.

Ock-Ja, L. "A Study on Deathbed and Death--Comparison of Clergyman with Medical Man." Taehan Kanho/Korean Nurse 21:2 (1982), 76-78.

Oppenheim, A.L. Ancient Mesopotamia--Portrait of a Dead Civilization. Chicago: University Press, 1964.

Osgood, N.J. "Suicide in the Elderly: Are We Heeding the Warnings." Postgraduate Medicine 72:2 (1982), 123-130.

Parkes, C.M. "Terminal Care: Evaluation of Effects in Surviving Family of Care Before and After Bereavement." Postgraduate Medical Journal 59 (June 1983), 73-78.

Peradotto, J. Classical Mythology. Chico, Calif.: Scholars, 1973.

Pettingill, W.L. Simple Studies in Matthew. Philadelphia: Philadelphia School of the Bible, n.d.

Piemme, J.A. "Death Education: A Different Approach." Oncology Nursing Forum 6:1 (1979), 4.

Pritchard, J., ed. Ancient Near Eastern Texts Relating to the Old Testament. Princeton, N.J.: Princeton University Press, 1969.

Rafferty, J.P. "The Personal Stress of Working with the Seriously Ill: Impact on the Caregiver." Progress in Clinical and Biological Research 121 (1983), 279-286.

Randolph-Flynn, P.A. Holistic Health--The Art and Science of Care. Bowie, Md.: Brady, 1980.

Rawlings, M. Before Death Comes. Nashville, Tenn.: Nelson, 1980.

Reed, E.L. Helping Children Cope with the Mystery of Death. Nashville, Tenn.: Abingdon Press, 1970.

Reicke, B. The Epistles of James, Peter, and Jude in the Anchor Bible, vol. 37, edited by W.F. Albright and D.N. Freedman. Garden City, N.Y.: Doubleday, 1964.

Richards, L. and P. Johnson. Death and the Caring Community. Portland, Ore.: Multnomah, 1980.

Ridderbos, H. Paul--An Outline of His Theology. Grand Rapids, Mich.: Eerdmans, 1975.

Robbins, J. "Careers--Care of the Dying: A Universal State." Nursing Mirror 154:13 (1982), 52.

Roberts, E. Heaven Has a Floor. New York: Damascus, 1979.

Robertson, J.M. Comfort. Wheaton, Ill.: Tyndale, 1982.

Rossman, P. Hospice. New York: Fawcett-Columbine, 1977.

Roskin, J. "Coping with Life Changes--A Preventive Social Work Approach." American Journal of Community Psychology 10:3 (1982), 331-340.

Rublee, D.A. and W.L. Yarber. "Instructional Units of Death Education: The Impact of the Amount of Classroom Time on Changes in Death Attitudes," Journal of School Health 53:7 (1983), 412-415.

Ryrie, C. The Ryrie Study Bible. Chicago: Moody, 1978.

Sachtleben, C.R. "The Role of Belief Systems in Cancer Therapy." Delaware Medical Journal 50:2 (1978), 71-72.

Sanders, J.R., T.E. Poole, and W.T. Rivero. "Death Anxiety Among the Elderly." Psychological Reports 46:1 (1980), 53-54.

Sanford, J.A. Evil--The Shadow Side of Reality. New York: Crossroads, 1984.

Sarna, N. Understanding Genesis. New York: Jewish Theological Seminary, 1966.

Saunders, C. "St. Christopher's Hospice." In E.S. Shneidman, Death: Current Perspectives, 2nd ed. Palo Alto, Calif.: Mayfield, 1976.

Schiff, H. The Bereaved Parent. New York: Penguin Books, 1977.

Schoenberg, B., A.C. Carr, D. Peretz, and A.H. Kutscher, eds. Loss and Grief: Psychological Management in Medical Practice. New York: Columbia University Press, 1970.

Schowalter, J., P. Patterson, M. Tallmer, A. Kutscher, S. Gullo, and D. Peretz, eds. The Child and Death. New York: Columbia University Press, 1983.

Schwarz, H. Beyond the Gates of Death. Minneapolis: Augsburg, 1981.

Scott, R.B.Y. Proverbs-Ecclesiastes in The Anchor Bible, vol. 18, edited by W.F. Albright and D.N. Freedman. Garden City, N.Y.: Doubleday, 1964.

Seybold, K. and U.B. Miller. Sickness and Healing, translated by D.W. Scott. Nashville, Tenn.: Abingdon Press, 1978.

Sheehy, G. Passages. New York: Bantam Books, 1977.

---. Pathfinders. New York: Bantam Books, 1982.

Shelly, J.A. The Spiritual Needs of Children. Downers Grove,
     Ill.: Intervarsity, 1982.

---. "Spiritual Care: Planting Seeds of Hope." Critical Care
     Update 9:12 (1982), 7-17.

Shipley, R. The Consumer's Guide to Death, Dying, and
     Bereavement. Palm Springs, Calif.: ETC, 1982.

Shneidman, E.S., ed. Death: Current Perspectives. Palo
     Alto, Calif.: Mayfield, 1980.

---, ed. Essays in Self-Destruction. New York: International
     Science Press, 1967.

Simmons, P.D. Birth and Death: Bioethical Decision-Making.
     Philadelphia: Westminster, 1983.

Southard, S. Training Church Members for Pastoral Care.
     Valley Forge, Pa.: Judson, 1982

Speiser, E. Genesis in The Anchor Bible, vol. 1, edited by
     W.F. Albright and D.N. Freedman. Garden City, N.Y.:
     Doubleday, 1974.

St. Clair, D. Psychic Healers. New York: Doubleday, 1963.

Stevens-Long, J. Adult Life--Developmental Processes. Palo
     Alto, Calif.: Mayfield, 1979.

Stone, H. The Caring Church. New York: Harper, 1983.

Swihart, P.J. The Edge of Death. Downers Grove, Ill.: In-
     tervarsity, 1978.

Swindoll, C. For Those Who Hurt. Portland, Ore.: Multnomah,
     1977.

Taylor, A.J. and A.G. Frazer. "The Stress of Post-Disaster
     Body Handling and Victim Identification Work." Journal
     of Human Stress 8:4 (1982), 4-12.

Thompson, I.E., C.P. Lowther, D. Doyle et al. "Learning
     About Death: A Project Report from the Edinburgh
     University Medical School." Journal of Medical Ethics
     7:2 (1981), 62-66.

Tousley, M.M. "The Use of Family Therapy in Terminal Ill-
     ness and Death." Journal of Psychosocial Nursing and
     Mental Health Services 20:1 (1982), 17-22.

Vander Lugt, H. The Art of Growing Old. Grand Rapids, Mich.: Radio Bible Class, 1980.

---. Light in the Valley. Grand Rapids, Mich.: Radio Bible Class, 1979.

Videka-Sherman, L. "Coping with the Death of a Child: A Study Over Time." American Journal of Orthopsychiatry 52:4 (1982), 688-698.

Wahl, P.R. "Therapeutic Relationships with the Elderly." Journal of Gerontological Nursing 6:5 (1980), 260-266.

Wass, H. et al. Death Education: An Annotated Resource Guide. New York: Hemisphere, 1980.

Weisman, A.D. and H.J. Sobel. "Coping with Cancer through Self-Instruction." Journal of Human Stress 5:1 (1979), 3-8.

Wenham, J. The Goodness of God. Downers Grove, Ill.: Intervarsity, 1974.

Wentz, F.K. The Layman's Role Today. New York: Abingdon Press, 1980.

Westermeyer, J. "Education and Counseling in Hospital Care." American Journal of Public Health 72:2, 127-128.

White, P. What's Happened to Auntie Jean? Glendale, Calif.: Regal, 1976.

Whitfield, J.M., R.E. Siegel, A.D. Glicken, R.J. Harmon, L.K. Powers, and E.J. Goldson. "The Application of Hospice Concepts to Neonatal Care." American Journal of Diseases of Children 136:5 (1982), 421-424.

Wilke, H. Creating the Caring Congregation: Guidelines for Ministering to the Handicapped. Nashville, Tenn.: Abingdon Press, 1980.

Winter, D. Hereafter. Wheaton, Ill.: Shaw, 1972.

Winton, R. "The Role of the Hospital Chaplain." The Medical Journal of Australia 1:13 (1982), 540.

Worden, J.W. and A.D. Weisman. "Do Cancer Patients Really Want Counseling?" General Hospital Psychiatry 2:2 (1980), 100-103.

Yancey, P. Where Is God When It Hurts? Grand Rapids,
    Mich.: Zondervan, 1979.

Zimring, J.G. "When Is the Physician 'Playing God'?" Journal
    of the American Geriatric Society 28:9 (1980), 419-21.

Zuesse, E.M. "The Absurdity of Ritual." Psychiatry 46
    (February 1983), 40-50.

6

Pastoral Care and Professional Burnout

D. T. Wessells, Jr.

Ministers, as do all helping professionals, face specific issues in their work that can produce high levels of stress. It is the goal of this chapter to identify those issues that are common to all helping professions. Having identified these issues, specific examples from pastoral care will be cited to aid in understanding the vocationally related stress experienced by the clergy. Finally, some solutions will be offered that can be developed into a training program to help ministers avoid professional burnout.

The determinants of job-related stress are based in two areas, one cognitive and the other interpersonal. The cognitive determinant has to do with how professionals define success and responsibility on the job. Professionals who are more focused on outcome and who hold themselves responsible for change in others are at higher risk of professional burnout than other workers. To clarify, helping professionals place their vocational energy into helping others to improve physically, emotionally, or spiritually. Many variables contribute to a "successful" or "unsuccessful" outcome of these efforts, most of which are beyond the influence of the helping professional. Unlike engineers or mechanics, who have more influence over work outcome, helping professionals are faced with the proposition of separating the effects of their efforts from all other influences on the client in order to judge their success. It is all too easy to deal with this complicated issue by becoming increasingly focused on outcome, that is, improvement in the client. Doing so gives one a sense of satisfaction and accomplishment when the client improves, but leads to frustration if the client's condition remains unchanged or deteriorates. For helping professionals, to take on this responsibility suggests that they are assuming responsibility for things beyond their control. In this light, helping professionals set unrealistic vocational expectations for themselves and program themselves to feel that they have failed if a client does not improve.

An alternative to focusing on outcome to evaluate job success requires changes in one's thinking. It is necessary to shift emphasis from the effects of one's work efforts to the quality of one's work efforts as a means of defining job success. As noted earlier, stress is generated by behaving on the job as though one can be responsible for things beyond one's control, particularly client outcome. Basing examination of the problem on what one can be responsible for enables the helping professional to set realistic job expectations. Specifically, defining job success by how one applies professional skills rather than on the outcome of their application is realistic. We are in control of and responsible for our own behavior on the job. In this regard, we can modify how we do our work to improve our skills, thus bringing job success more within our control. Being able to obtain success on the job more readily leads to satisfaction and reduces the stress inherent in failures, over which we have only partial control. A concern often expressed in response to these notions is the effect on outcome if one chooses not to focus on it. In the long term, to focus on the process of work rather than the outcome only serves to improve the outcome.

The second determinant of job-related stress is interpersonal in nature. This aspect is difficult to describe. The key here has to do with how one handles the tension that develops in working relationships. These relationships can be between professional and client, professional and professional, or any other combination of individuals. A common pattern that leads to increased stressfulness in the work environment occurs when one person is upset by a second person and turns to a third party to dissipate the tension. In this instance, emotional distance develops between the first two persons and closeness develops between the first person and the confidant. Each time the first person encounters the same problem and handles it in the same manner, the stress in the work environment is increased. What this pattern accomplishes is the perpetuation of unsatisfactory work relationships.

To explain this pattern, an example may be helpful. A minister receives a call from an unusually demanding parishioner, who requests commitments from the minister with which the minister complies, but resentfully. After the call, the minister turns to his secretary and complains about his overcrowded schedule. The secretary responds by offering the minister support and understanding, which enables the minister to begin to feel better. The incident has fostered a sense of closeness between the minister and his secretary. In addition, it has caused the secretary to begin to worry about how her boss does not take good care of himself. The following week, the same parishioner calls with more demands. This reactivates the pattern and adds to the anxiety being contained between the minister and his secretary.

By using the secretary as the solution for handling his anxiety, the minister cuts himself off from developing new behaviors to deal with the stress of encountering demanding parishioners. A further complication occurs between the minister and secretary. With her focus on her boss as an unfortunate and overworked man, she is not likely to bring up issues with him that bother her because she does not want to add to his distress. Thus, the pattern also masks potential tensions in their relationship. In this example of coping with stressful encounters, the anxiety-producing interpersonal encounters are perpetuated and add to the stressfulness of the work environment.

To counter this unhealthy interpersonal pattern, ministers must learn to handle tension in the relationships that generate it. To do this, they must begin by evaluating how they define their responsibility to their parishioners. In the example cited, it is likely that the minister feels and acts as though he is responsible for keeping his parishioners happy. He fails to consider the unreasonableness of some requests of the personal imposition he faces in attempting to meet parishioners' needs. He is likely to be most aware of his sense of frustration or failure if he is unable to please a parishioner. It is obvious that no matter how hard he may try, it is impossible to please everybody. Therefore, the minister would be well advised to redefine his responsibility to his parishioners in realistic, obtainable terms. In doing so, he should balance that responsibility with an awareness of the need to take good care of himself, spiritually, physically, and emotionally, so that he can be an effective minister to his parishioners.

With this redefinition, the minister can consider alternative approaches to stressful encounters, and ones that do not necessarily require pleasing parishioners. The minister would be best served by putting his energy into developing techniques to handle demanding parishioners. He may want to use his secretary or others for emotional support so that he can begin to develop creative ways of setting limits on demands for his time. This will become easier to do when the minister gives up trying to be responsible for his parishioners' happiness. Accordingly, the secretary is not viewed as the solution, but only a resource to provide support for the minister in developing solutions. In the short run, this may add anxiety to the work environment; however, with increased demonstration of the minister's ability to handle these problems, the anxiety will lessen. This form of coping with stressful interpersonal encounters reduces the stressfulness of the work environment and the likelihood of burnout.

Having explored the determinants of job stress in theoretical terms, attention will now be turned to specific issues identified by ministers as relating to the stressfulness of their work. The issues to be discussed were drawn from a questionnaire and personal interviews. The most prevalent sources of job stress identified by ministers were interpersonal issues related to limit setting in relation to parishioners' demands. Secondary to this were mediation issues, especially if anger was expressed.

In reviewing the questionnaires for items that addressed responsibility themes, it was evident that respondents, for the most part, held themselves responsible for things beyond their control. Common responses to the question of how they defined success were "having been helpful to others," "seeing growth in parishioners," and "receiving compliments from parishioners." In turn, failure was experienced "if I wasn't helpful," "if the church hierarchy frustrated my efforts," "if I failed to say no to parishioners who could be served by others," and "if I did not please parishioners." These responses suggest that ministers hold themselves responsible for change in others and for decision making, even when they possess only partial power to make those decisions. Although these goals are worthy of attainment, in each case the minister responding had only limited ability to realize the goal. Hence, these goals were unrealistic as measures of job success and responsibility for the ministers. Few responses focused on how well the ministers acted in their role as helpers (e.g., "I am successful when I can be with a disturbed parishioner and remain detached enough to be a good listener, yet involved enough to be empathetic"). Pastors who operate in this manner are likely to effect positive outcomes, but their success is based on their own behavior rather than on changes in their parishioners.

The respondent noted above who failed by not saying "no" appears to be having difficulty in setting realistic limits. Two other respondents, addressing the theme of responsibility to parishioners, defined their role in pastoral care as that of "facilitator." These respondents used this posture to remove themselves from being responsible for meeting parishioners' needs, instead assuming responsibility for assisting parishioners in meeting their own needs. Although this appears to be a change in semantics rather than a change in definition of job role, the implications are significant. An example can be used to illustrate the difference. As a facilitator, a minister can tend to the emotional needs of a parishioner by arranging an interview with a mental-health professional. Whether or not the parishioner follows through with the referral is the responsibility and choice of the parishioner. The minister has behaved responsibly in his facilitator role by making the referral. Conversely, ministers who define their role as meeting the needs of parishioners (that is, pleasing them) may attempt to provide direct assistance for the emotional needs of a disturbed parishioner. In the example given, the minister can find himself confronting a problem for which he may not be suitably trained; at best, he will invest large amounts of time in efforts that pertain only peripherally to his main job functions. Therefore, by assuming the facilitator role, these respondents are undoubtedly able to define their role in a way that better meets their needs. First, as ministers, they are able to function as facilitators with no need for specialized expertise, and consequently can readily experience success in the role. Second, by not delivering direct services, these ministers are able to lessen the demands on their already busy schedules while offering parishioners avenues to resolve their problems.

A review of the questionnaire items examining the interpersonal aspects of the ministry indicated that most respondents cope by containing their frustrating feelings and by distancing themselves from the sources of frustration. As in the example cited earlier, involving the hypothetical minister and his secretary, those respondents who reported that they seek support from others appear to use the support to help them avoid confronting stressful situations.

Common responses to the item "When you feel upset or depressed, what do you do to cope?" included "take a trip," "meditate," "sail," and other activities designed to remove their focus from their feelings. Respondents who reported that they seek support from others identified the supportive others as wife or a colleague. It is worth noting that those who reported seeking support were in the minority of the respondents. The questionnaire did not adequately assess how these ministers use their supportive relationships. However, there was no suggestion in the responses that the supportive relationships are used to help the ministers confront and find solutions to the stressful situation in question. One might suspect that respondents either contained their anxiety within themselves or externalized it in a relationship system, as in the case of the imaginary minister who complained to his secretary and did nothing to deal with the persistent parishioner.

To summarize the questionnaire findings, most respondents reported operating in an overly responsible posture in significant areas of their professional lives. This behavior will continue to contribute to the frustration and stress they experience as ministers. Second, respondents seldom reported using the anxiety inherent in their work to motivate them to take actions designed to alleviate or lessen stressful situations. By and large the responses indicated that they either contained their anxiety or externalized it into either the home or the professional environment. In the latter case, externalization may add to the stressfulness of either the home or work environment, since it was not augmented by efforts to confront the problem constructively.

The results of this survey, although far from scientific, seem to substantiate the concepts outlined earlier concerning the etiology of work-related stress. What follows is an outline of those areas seen as important in the training of ministers to cope better with work-related stress.

Training to cope emotionally with work stressors is best accomplished in a group setting. This enables participants to gain emotional support, as well as to practice new behaviors that are imparted in the training. One of the early tasks of the group is to deal with developing a set of realistic work expectations. Using the concept of over- and underresponsibility, the group can assist participants in defining for themselves a responsible position to take in numerous problem work areas. A second focus for this training is on principles of interpersonal communication. Specifically, a concept drawn from Bowen systems theory, called triangling, is useful (Bowen 1978). This concept enables participants to understand different patterns of communication in calm and stressful interpersonal environments. Such understanding is critical in developing means of confronting work stressors in a positive, creative manner. Finally, assertiveness and communication issues need be addressed to enable participants to alter their behaviors in constructive ways to cope with stressful interpersonal encounters.

In closing, some suggestions may be useful in implementing this training model. Training of this nature is best conducted by a trained mental-health practitioner who has an interest in the areas noted above. Further, the training is designed to be long-term. Such a training group could easily meet on a weekly basis for a year or more. Once a group of this nature gels, the organization of the group reinforces its use as an appropriate support medium to help ministers effectively handle work-related stress. Through this vehicle, professional fulfillment becomes a realistic goal for those motivated to become involved in the training experience.

REFERENCE

Bowen, M. Family Therapy in Clinical Practice. New York: Jason Aronson, 1978.

Part II

Death and Dying

7

A Holistic Model for Care of the Dying

Steven A. Moss

It can be said that the modern discipline of thanatology began in 1969, with the publication of On Death and Dying by Kübler-Ross. Her book presented to both the professional and lay communities a clearer understanding of what may happen psychosocially to dying people. The insights into the process of dying, which she delineated in five stages, sensitized our society "to the human needs of the patient who wants to be treated not as a clinical specimen but as a person" (Kübler-Ross 1969).

In the decade and a half since Kübler-Ross's original work, the major criticism of her book has focused on the use of the word "stages." It has been pointed out by many that dying cannot be staged. This is especially true if the effect of staging is to assume a priori that every dying person will go through these stages in the order presented by Kübler-Ross, and that the goal of those who care for the dying is to bring them to that last stage of acceptance before death comes. The critics see this view of staging as too categorical, tending to treat the person who is dying more like an object to be staged than as a person to be encountered as a human being.

Kübler-Ross (1974) answered these critics when she wrote:

I think it is important to emphasize that our goal should not be to help people through the five stages and reach the stage of acceptance. The outline of these five stages is only the common denominator that we found in most of our terminally ill patients. Many do not flow from stage one to five in a chronological order, and this is totally irrelevant to their well-

being. Our goal should be to elicit the patient's needs, to find out where he is.

The stages should, therefore, be seen as giving direction and guidance to care of the dying. They are a guide to
comprehending how the dying react to their dying. The
stages of denial and isolation, anger, bargaining, depression,
and acceptance are exhibited by the dying in many ways:
verbally and nonverbally, psychologically, socially, intellec-
tually, and spiritually. Those who care for the dying will
determine the stage they are in by viewing and analyzing
their behavior. Such determinations will be useful for them
in giving the appropriate means of support and attention.

In an attempt to understand the process of dying and
how care-givers can be helpful to the dying in that process,
Pattison (1977) described the living-dying interval. According to Pattison, there is a dying trajectory that is composed
of a potential death trajectory and an actual death trajectory.
The potential death trajectory is always present in people's
lives, either consciously or subconsciously.

All of us live with the potential for death at any moment. All of us project ahead a trajectory of our life. That is,
we anticipate a certain life-span within which we arrange our
activities and plan our lives (Pattison 1977). Whether by illness or accident, the potential death trajectory can become
actual. With this "crisis of knowledge of death," the living-
dying interval begins. With the crisis of knowledge, an acute
crisis phase begins and is accompanied by peak anxiety. A
second phase, which Pattison calls "chronic living-dying,"
leads to the terminal phase, which ends with the point of
death.

Pattison's dying trajectory uses a descriptive diagrammatical model to see the dying process most clearly. The
living-dying interval is placed on a time line, with each time
segment of this interval in a person's life clearly delineated
as part of this dying process. This dying trajectory and
Pattison's diagrammatical model of it are more descriptive and
less prescriptive than Kübler-Ross's initial concept of stages.
They allow the care-giver to see this process as a whole in
terms of a continuum of time in a person's life. The concept
of a dying trajectory implies flow and movement within life's
experiences, including that of dying.

Within the living-dying interval, Pattison (1977) aptly
described all aspects of the dying person's life and environmental structure, including a diagramming of the biological,
psychological, physical, and sociological death along the time
line of the terminal phase. Such descriptive diagramming of
the dying process allows care-givers to see the whole of a
dying person's experiences. This diagramming can also be
used as a tool by those who work with the dying, allowing

them to see clearly where a dying person is on the time line.
With this knowledge and understanding, care-givers can adjust their methods of care and intervention and can involve
other professionals in that care as seems appropriate to give
the best care possible. This descriptive diagramming can also
be used as a post-mortem technique, allowing care-givers to
learn how and in what ways it might be possible to help others who are dying.

Pattison's living-dying interval and its diagrams fit in
well with the current concept of holistic treatment. As an
understanding spreads throughout the sciences and humani-
ties that "an entity is greater in its wholeness than the sum
of its parts, a new plateau of existence is reached when this
new wholeness is obtained." Thus, health care now looks to
treat an integrated unity of mind, body, and spirit.

Pattison's descriptive diagrams are limited in that they
are one-dimensional. They use a linear time line in their descriptive approach and, therefore, do not present a total,
holistic picture of all of the components of the dying process
as these constantly interact in an almost three-dimensional
way.

A true holistic model must be three-dimensional, reflecting the various dimensions of the dying person's life. These
are: (1) the inner dimension, including psychological, emotional, intellectual, and spiritual components; (2) the environmental dimension, including family and community components;
and (3) the physical dimension, including past physical ailments that can affect the present condition, as well as present ailments, pains, and so on. Each dimension should be di-
agrammed as a circle with its various components moving
along the circumference. In other words, the diagram is made
up of three wheels, each representing a dimension of the
person's dying. The area of intersection of the circles represents the person at a given moment along the living-dying
interval time line. All three circles are in movement, just as
a person's inner, environmental, and physical dimensions are
always in movement. All these circles move simultaneously
along Pattison's living-dying interval, giving a holistic picture of the dying process. As the circles move along the time
line they become smaller as the moment of death approaches,
as the person's world and experiences become smaller.

This holistic model of the dying process gives a true
picture of the dying person along the living-dying interval.
Such a model is extremely useful for post-mortem analysis,
but, even more importantly, it enables care-givers to see how
they can best help the dying person. A day-to-day log using
this diagram can be kept. In this way, movements of the circles can be seen and ways of helping the dying can be pre-
dicted and adjusted. Care-givers can visualize all components
of the dying person's life in order to decide what to do and

to determine what other professionals are necessary to meet the needs brought to light by the diagram.

Holistic care of the dying needs a holistic model that allows those who care for the dying to view the dying person's life on all levels. Such a view must contribute to optimal loving care of the dying. It must contribute to enhanced care of the dying, whereby they will be treated as persons and not as objects. It is this kind of care that they so sorely need.

REFERENCES

Heller, Z.I. "The Jewish View of Death: Guidelines for Dying." In E. Kübler-Ross, ed., Death, The Final Stage of Growth, p. 39. Englewood Cliffs, N.J.: Prentice-Hall, 1975.

Kübler-Ross, E. On Death and Dying. New York: Macmillan, 1969.

---. Questions and Answers on Death and Dying, p. 71. New York: Macmillan, 1974.

Pattison, E.M. The Experience of Dying, p. 44. Englewood Cliffs, N.J.: Prentice-Hall, 1977.

8

Caring for the Dying

William B. Smith

In focusing on pastoral care issues in experiences of
loss, death, and bereavement, I offer a caution. I don't do
so to dampen the enthusiasm or professionalism of anyone,
but rather to trigger, I hope, a little bit of realism. St. Paul
concludes the fifteenth chapter of his first Letter to the
Corinthians with a triumphant, faith-filled affirmation of continuity between this life and the next. He says that "Death
is swallowed up in victory" (1 Cor. 15:54), and asks "O
death where is your victory? O death where is your sting?"
(1 Cor. 15:55). He concludes: "Be steadfast and preserving.
. . . You know that your toil is not in vain when it is done
in the Lord" (1 Cor. 15:58). I accept and share the same
faith, but I wonder today whether death is being swallowed
up in jargon. Many in our society seem not to ask Paul's
questions, but "O death where is your definition? O death
where is your uniform statute?" Some Christians forget the
context of Paul's questions. In First Corinthians (15:5), he
says, "Now I am going to tell you a mystery." A mystery--
not a game plan, a legislative tactic, a social movement, or
a trend--but a mystery.

I offer this caution because I suspect that so much
emphasis has been placed on how natural a part of life death
is that the good and needed effort to talk about, even to
mention death may well have been all too successful. Any
randomly selected group of 30 Ph.D.s or their equivalent
might well explain how natural a part of life death is. However, any 30 million people from elsewhere would not share
that kind of academic temperateness about death.

In a way, I am repeating the quiet caution long since
raised by Ramsey (1974) and Kass (1974) that "death-with-
dignity" is too readily promoted and too readily accepted. To
insist, as some do, that death is quite as natural an occur-

rence as birth smacks, at times, of soap-opera stuff. I do not
doubt that death can be so defined, but simply question how
often that definition is readily accepted or realized. Obviously, no one makes a case for "indignity," but I share with
Ramsey (1974) the fear that some people romantically invest
death with a bogus dignity that is really a cover-up, if not
a hindrance to proper care of the dying.

Dignity in the face of death cannot be created extrinsically; it can neither be invented by law nor programmed by
committee. If it exists at all, it is intrinsic, internal to the
person who so approaches death. Personally, I favor the notion of death with dignity, properly defined as living with
dignity even when one is dying. However, I suspect that
death with dignity is about as available as life with dignity,
which is not and never has been available to all.

For most people, death represents and is the ultimate
in the unknown. For that reason alone, it truly frightens
most people. Even for a Christian who looks forward to eternal life, and who believes, as I do, again with St. Paul, that
I would "rather be away from the body and at home with the
Lord" (2 Cor. 5:8), death may hold no fear, but the prospect of going through the process of dying is terrifying
(Koop 1976).

Even separation that is real is a loss that is real. Most
often it is, I think, loss and separation that are feared. We
fear the loss of employment, the loss of security and, indeed,
any move or transfer from the known to the unknown, from
connections to the apparent absence of connections. All of
these are approached with some trepidation. Death is one
cause of such loss and separation that is so feared.

Some of the reasons that are mentioned in favor of
legislation for so-called living wills and natural-death acts--
legislation I consider unnecessary and dangerous--nonetheless
involve fears that do surround either death or the dying
process. These fears need attention and resolution which, in
my judgment, legislation cannot and will not accomplish.

Certainly, we can all understand the concern or distress that some feel about excessive technological intervention
in the dying process. Next, we can all appreciate the fear of
the all-too-frequent control of that process by professionals
rather than by patients and their families. Also, in our highly litigious society, we can appreciate the fear of malpractice
suits among physicians and hospital administrators. However,
none of these difficulties will be solved by additional and
unnecessary legislation. Although the compassion that is said
to motivate such proposals is noteworthy, it is unfortunately
true that we cannot legislate compassion, any more than we
can legislate trust. Indeed, the superabundance of laws is
quiet testimony to the fact that we really don't trust each
other very much any more.

The foregoing is offered as cautions; the following I offer as comment by way of example. I am a director, a member
of the board of trustees of Calvary Hospital in the Bronx,
New York, an institution dedicated exclusively to the care of
patients who have advanced cancer. Calvary Hospital is a
unique hospital; we are, half-jokingly and half-not, the UN
hospice. Some central elements of the Calvary philosophy, as
well as the special place it gives to pastoral care, may provide useful points for reflection.

One key element of Calvary's philosophy is a policy of
nonabandonment. We know there is no cure for our patients,
but we promise all of them humane care, always. When there
is no cure, we still provide humane care. That principled
commitment is a source of relief to a great number of people,
both patients and their families.

When death is inevitable or even imminent, many people
have a real fear of being abandoned. Thus, at Calvary, we
take some effort to address that concern clearly and fully.
As you walk into the main lobby of our hospital, there is a
large donor wall for all to see and read. The words inscribed
on that wall are taken from the book of Genesis. In two
verses they say what the hospital has been committed to for
the last 80 years:

> I will never leave you until I have done what
> I have promised you [Gen. 28:15, and]
> This is none other than the House of God,
> and this is the Gate of Heaven [Gen. 28:17].

"I will never leave you until I have done what I have prom-
ised you." That is our promise to our patients whom we cannot cure, but for whom we can and do care. It is our promise not to abandon them. That promise is a great help to a
great many.

The pastoral care department at Calvary Hospital is a
core component of the hospital, not just an appendage. As a
religiously affiliated institution, we are open to all, but we
will yield to none that loss, death, and bereavement are
simply technical aspects of a technical question called death.

Just as our philosophy requires us not to abandon
patients, so it also requires us not to abandon our commitment to the whole patient--body, mind, soul, and spirit. In
our philosophy, human life is not merely the sum total of
biological parts and biochemical processes. Human life and,
thereby, human worth include the human soul and the human
spirit as well--these, too, we commit ourselves not to abandon.

It is this value-rooted vision that prompts our pastoral-
care department to attend to patients and their families as
death approaches, when death occurs, and after death, in

funeral services for all faiths. We find that this policy of not abandoning either patients or their families is a great relief and comfort throughout loss, death, and bereavement.

The vision of Calvary Hospital is linked securely to the values it proclaims and sustains: the inherent dignity of every human life. In that vision, Calvary sees chronic illness and death as a transition and not an extinction. People should never be narrowly reduced to the diseases that afflict them, however serious those diseases or however complicated the care required. Thus, again, we aim to serve the whole patient, and that service extends beyond the technical delivery of bodily sustenance and somatic relief to include the care and service of the mind, the soul, the spirit.

The fact of advanced cancer necessarily involves the consideration of death. Whether this is a proximate or a remote fact, we still offer humane care when there is no cure. Chronic illness and death are not like other life events; they are singular, not at all routine. Sometimes they are feared, largely because they have not been personally experienced; but within the perspective of life's true worth and purpose, they are best served by a full response to the whole person --body, mind, soul, and spirit.

The experience of Calvary Hospital may be almost unique in matters of loss, death, and bereavement. Certainly Calvary is not unique in its willingness to learn from others to improve its own continuing experience or in its willingness to share with others the experience we have gleaned from our own practice as a working and practical model for pastoral care in loss, death, and bereavement.

REFERENCES

Kass, L.R. "Averting One's Eyes or Facing the Music? On Dignity in Death." Hastings Center Studies 2:2 (1974), 67-80.

Koop, C.E. The Right to Live, the Right to Die, p. 83. Wheaton, Ill.: Tyndale House, 1976.

"Living Will Legislation Opposed." Origins 9:40 (March 20, 1980):pp. 650-651.

Ramsey, P. "The Indignity of Death and Dignity." Hastings Center Studies 2:2 (1974), 47-62.

9

Death: A Theological Reappraisal

Thomas McGowan

Until very recently, Western society has kept the subject of death on the fringes of human consciousness and
polite conversation by the strictly applied defenses of self-
deception and the use of elaborate euphemisms. Just as the
Victorian age found it necessary to deal with sex pornograph-
ically, so the twentieth century has resorted to treating
death in a psychologically unhealthy way. Both sex and death
have been shunted into the dark corners of existence instead
of being faced as valid human experiences. Lately, however,
there seems to be evidence of a healthy attempt to confront
death as a reality and to position it within the total context
of life. This new consciousness has shown itself surprisingly
among students in colleges all across the country, who have
shown a sustained interest in courses on death. For example,
Manhattan College (New York City) has, for the past decade,
offered a course entitled "Death as a Fact of Life," and each
semester more than 100 students have filled its three sections.
    Although some students begin the course thinking that
it will answer their most troubling questions about death,
they are quickly brought to accept the more realistic goal of
trying to understand the feelings and experiences of dying
people, the moral decisions often forced upon them in their
dying, the grief process, the social rituals connected with
dying and death, and the hopes for life after death. All of
this is approached in an interdisciplinary fashion, but since
this is a course within the religious studies department,
there is a special focus on the theological understanding of
death. This chapter will be limited to a brief account of this
kind of theological effort to describe death.
    When first asked to define death, most students identi-
fy with one of three possible attitudes: that death is natural
and, as such, requires no explanation; that death is unnatu-

ral and thus is a violation of what it means to be human; and finally, that death is somehow the very act that makes us human. I shall look briefly at the first two of these attitudes and then try to show how Christian theology interprets death as a humanizing event.

The argument that death is an integral part of what constitutes "nature" is perhaps best illustrated in Freud's (1975) analysis of the death instinct. Freud's premise is that the essence of reality is chaos and not the "oceanic feeling" or sense of oneness and community that the infantile ego seeks. The universe is ultimately disordered, unharmonious, and diffuse. Since Freud sees instinct as "an urge inherent in organic life to restore an earlier state of things," it leads inevitably to a return to that initial condition of simplicity and separateness. The highly complex reality called human life falls back to its original inorganic state. The conclusion is evident: since everything living dies for internal reasons, death is the most natural of human events.

De Beauvoir, however is not satisfied with such an explanation. She sees life as a series of unanswered questions and death as the stumbling block that makes these questions unanswerable. In A Very Easy Death (1966) she denies that there is any such thing as a natural death. Since a human's very presence calls the whole world into question, the individual is not limited even by death. According to de Beauvoir's view, death is always an "accident" and an "unjustifiable violation." A similar sense of frustration is expressed by Dylan Thomas (1971):

> Do not go gentle into that good night.
> Old age should burn and rave at close of day;
> Rage, rage against the dying of the light.

In this view, death is the enigma that infests life with the germs of absurdity. Human existence must be wrenched out of the simply natural if it is to have any unique value. But death always lurks as the enemy, always casts doubts on whatever humans accomplish, always seems to win out over life at the end. This is an intolerable situation that we must rail against if we are to maintain any semblance of humanity in the face of death.

Perhaps the posture of Simone de Beauvoir and Dylan Thomas reflects the existentialist retreat in which the individual soon discovers that the self, the singular "I," cannot cope with death alone. An "otherness" or a "you" seems to be necessary to people if they are to be redeemed in death by discovering their real destiny. Tolstoy's classic story, "The Death of Ivan Ilyich," illustrates very well the necessity of human relations in making death a fulfilling rather than a horrifying experience. Tolstoy does not dismiss death by appealing to facile Christian optimism; rather, he reconciles himself to it by taking to heart the religious maxim that it is only in losing the self that one can find the self. This can be achieved most authentically, says Tolstoy, in the very act of dying. Ivan Ilyich has been caught up in the web of secrecy with which society hides both life and death. It is only through the death-affirming peasant Gerasim that Ivan comes to recognize that death is not an intruder that attacks from without, but instead the creative act of coming to one's self by letting go. When he does this, all that has been oppressing him drops away--fear, pain, even death itself--and only the unchanging truth of what it is to be human remains.

Tolstoy's thought serves as a model for a contemporary reinterpretation of traditional Christian doctrinal statements about death. People are not defined in terms of what they share with animals and plants but in terms of what is utterly distinctive to humanity. Therefore, when Christian faith proclaims the universality of death, it is not stating a self-evident biological fact, but rather something proper to human beings and to their relationship with God. It is only in death that people are full, free, spiritual beings, because only then can they most meaningfully choose to be so. If people never died, if they were doomed to an unending life of temporariness and incompletion, their freedom and their very humanity would be crippled. Why should they plan anything? Why undertake anything?

Only those who must die are capable of truly loving life, of running risks, of believing in the future. The great insight of Christian people when they proclaim mortality is that death is a gift and not a curse: it is the ultimate boundary of human potentialities. Of course, Christian theology also says that death is the consequence of sin. This is not a claim, however, that the first person would not have died biologically. What it seems to say is that although death should have been the pure act of self-affirmation, it has become a thing of suffering and fear. So death is the "result of sin" in the sense that it is seen as destruction from without instead of creation from within.

Another doctrine that needs reexamination is the belief that death somehow marks the absolute end of individuals' moral lives and locks them into an unalterable state in heaven or hell. Usually this notion carries images of death as a stalking antagonist, waiting to pounce on the unwary and hold them forever in bliss or woe. But, once again, if death is seen as a process of self-creation, then such a view is absurd. Could not the Christian community be saying, rather, that death gives people the opportunity to perform their first completely personal act? All other human acts are characterized by the essential temporariness of our existence; because they are time-bound, they are always liable to revision. Death faces no time, however, and so poses the opportunity for the complete awakening of consciousness, for freedom, for total encounter with God, for the final decision about human destiny. This is not to say that there can be no further growth in personhood, but only that once a completely free choice has been made we would never again freely want to alter it. Such an interpretation of this doctrine is consistent in seeing death as an active consummation from within, a growing up, the achieving of the total self.

When Christian faith defines death as a separation of body and soul, it should be remembered that this theological construct is not in itself the object of faith, but rather the effort of believing people to speak meaningfully about the eschatological mysteries. Hellenistic philosophy, not biblical religion, was the agent that split the human person into two parts and, in a sense, denied death by claiming immortality of the spirit. The Greeks viewed death as a kind of escape of the person from the imprisonment of the body. It is not surprising, therefore, that Paul was scoffed at by the Athenians for preaching resurrection, a doctrine that faces squarely the nonbeing of death and yet hopes for the gift of new creation. The Christian belief in resurrection is different from the philosophical belief in an immortal soul. In fact, facile denial of the radicalness of death by overemphasizing the belief that the soul never dies does a disservice to Christian faith. What can resurrection possibly mean if death is so glibly brushed aside? Surely resurrection involves more than the mere resuscitation of the body for an eventual reunion with the soul; it must point to something completely new and unmerited in human destiny.

Perhaps it would be beneficial to restate the "separation of body and soul" formula in terms of a binding together rather than of dividing. Traditional norms of behavior insist on preserving the ego as a separate entity to be guarded and preserved even while it enters into necessary relationships with other independent egos. Society frequently judges sanity to rest on the individual's capacity to adapt to the external world and to avoid, as much as possible, any personal direct awareness of the inner world. People are said to be insane when their self-consciousness slips into a larger context of consciousness and they lose their sense of self-identity. Yet all religious traditions speak of reality precisely in terms of such a loss of self as the necessary means to discover the true self. Through the death of the false self, which has betrayed its nature by completely adjusting to a universe alienated from God, the true or inner self can emerge as servant of the divine. Some theologians suggest that the answer to this dilemma lies in an interpretation of death that sees the soul as entering into some deeper, all-embracing openness to the universe and to God. The pouring out of self at death

leads to a new "pan-cosmic" reality that is not too foriegn to
the concept of union with the "All," the state of Nirvana
presented in some of the Eastern religions.

A final doctrine that deserves to be looked at in light
of this personalist approach concerns the death of Jesus
Christ as the central act of human salvation. The Christian
church has long labored to give adequate expression to the
mission of Jesus and, in the course of its history, has evolved
various atonement theories. Western theology, however,
has been dominated by St. Anselm's eleventh-century argument that Jesus' death supplied the satisfaction needed to
placate a God made angry by sin. When Anselm asked why
God became man, he answered rather legalistically that only
the God-man could make up for sin; the sacrifice and death
of the incarnate Son were demanded in justice to the Father.
However, this thesis is distasteful to contemporary believers,
steeped in the language and sentiment of an I-Thou encounter between God and man. The God who loves us and makes
covenants with us transcends the ogre who demands his
pound of flesh in retribution for sin. Anselm's view cheapens
the Christ-event, the great revelatory outpouring of God into
his creation, by limiting it to its soteriological aspects. A reinterpretation of the death of Jesus is therefore necessary if
we are to go beyond Anselm's legalisms to a more relational
and revelational understanding of the mystery.

If Jesus' death is seen as his final act of self-validation,
then perhaps the doctrine of redemption may regain its vitality for today's believer. Contemporary theology must first of
all demythologize the account of a descending God who assumed human flesh in order to pay back in his own blood for
man's offenses. A more meaningful paradigm might be that of
Ralph Waldo Emerson, who described Jesus Christ as the man
who recognized the integral relationship of God to man, and
who could therefore truly proclaim his own divinity. Emerson
held that all human beings are called to follow Jesus in the
same self-discovery. Salvation, in this sense of touching the
ultimate in human possibilities, cannot be limited to any one
event, but must involve a long process of revelation. Jesus'
death was redemptive, therefore, in that it was the final
human and, indeed, "humanizing" act of his life. In death,
Jesus fully discovered who he was and entered into an un-
restricted relationship with the whole world. His body was
shattered and he was poured out so as to be present to all
creation in his death. Resurrection, an inseparable dimension
of these mysteries, may be seen as this continued presence
of Jesus and as the pledge that we also will pass with Jesus
through death to our own salvation. The joyous claim of Eas-
ter, then, is that death is not the end of human personality.

In Christian practice, this passage through death to
new being is ritualized in sacrament. Baptism, for instance,

signifies the end of our previous existence and our opening
to a new identity in Christ. Unfortunately, contemporary custom often shifts the symbolism from this death-life cycle to
one of washing, but the ancient rubric clearly intended that
catechumens be divested of their old personalities by plung-
ing into the water and symbolically dying with Christ. Like
Christ, they then rise, put on new clothes, take new names,
and assume the new dignity of "Christed" persons. Similarly,
the Eucharist celebrates, in the breaking of the bread, the
reconciling power of the death of Christ for the church. The
alienated, fearful people who symbolically die with Christ rise
up as a unified community of Christians, a rebuilt body of
Christ.

Such rites of passage depict death as a part of the law
of human growth. If individuals are to come to full maturity,
they must consciously and freely relinquish the old, as the
baby leaves the womb, in order to take on the new being
that is offered. Of course, change is always feared because
it is a plunge into the unknown. Christians are no more secure in the face of death than anyone else, yet their faith is
that death is indeed a creative and humanizing event. Christians are willing to leap into this last unknown in the belief
that they will be grasped by Christ.

REFERENCES

de Beauvoir, S. A Very Easy Death, translated by P. O'Brien.
    New York: G.P. Putnam's Sons, 1966.

Freud, S. Beyond the Pleasure Principle, edited by J.
    Strachey. New York: W.W. Norton, 1975.

Thomas, D. "Do Not Go Gentle Into That Good Night." The
    Collected Poems. New York: New Directions, 1971.

Tolstoy, L. The Death of Ivan Ilyich and Other Stories. New
    York: New American Library, 1960.

10

The Interface of Psychiatry and Religion

Robert H. Springer

Three experiences have taught me more about death and bereavement than I had known before in all my years of clerical ministry. The first experience involved a homosexual man dying in the arms of his lover. The second involved a cancer victim leaving a wife and three-year-old child. In the third instance, a man dying of cancer could not face death because he knew his family still needed him.

All three of these persons exhibited diverse manifestations of the fear of death. Two instances required instructing the families to let go of their departing member. Underlying the experience of all three was a religious belief system: God is the Lord of life and death; you may not die until God comes for you. The theology supporting this belief needed reinterpretation for the dying and for the families.

Harry (I call him this to preserve confidentiality) was in the final weeks of life with cancer that gnawed at his vitals. His grown daughter and son attended him lovingly around the clock, assisted by a faithful friend who took time off from work to be with Harry when they needed rest. Harry was restless, struggling constantly to get out of bed and stand on his feet. He was so debilitated that those caring for him were afraid that he would fall through the hospital window. His mind alternated between reality and illusion. As his daughter confided to me, his worst pain was the thought, "My family still needs me." The thought had a real basis in the fact that one of his sons was having serious problems in straightening out his life.

On my second visit I spoke with him alone, hoping my words were penetrating his dazed and obsessed mind.

Harry, it's all right to go now. God is waiting
for you. . . . Don't worry about your family.

We will take care of your son. You have done
all that God expects you to do. It's time for you
to go to Jesus. And, Harry, it's all right to let
go when you want to. You don't have to struggle
endlessly.

When I phoned the family the next day, I learned that Harry,
who had been expected to hold on doggedly for days, had
passed on peacefully the night before. He had needed the
church to tell him it was all right for him to go and that he
might choose the time.

James, a 40-year-old, homosexual Catholic, had been
brought back from the hospital by Charles, his lover, to die
at home. Charles had phoned me: "Please come, Father, but
don't disturb him with last rites. He's not near death yet.
Just say some prayers and bring Communion." Sensing ambiguity in the caller's message, I went prepared for anything.
When I arrived, I found James sitting up in bed, his voice
quite strong, his mind clear. We exchanged greetings, and
then, unexpectedly, he said: "I'm glad you came. I haven't
got long to live." I asked, "How do you feel about that?"
"Not very good. I'm disappointed." "You mean disappointed
with God for not letting you live longer?" "Yes, I had hoped
to have so much more of life." He spoke on about his disappointment. He ended by saying, with conviction, "But then,
I've packed more into 40 years than most people do into 80."
I had never witnessed such quick transition through Kübler-
Ross's stages. Or had he been at stage four all along and
Charles, who held him in his arms, in stage one? More likely
the latter, I thought.

Yes, James wanted confession, which I heard in private.
James then requested Communion. Charles brought bread and
wine from the kitchen and other members of the household
converged. We did the Mass liturgy with bread and book lying on James's bed. I sensed faith all around, and felt gratitude that God had not abandoned these people in the hour of
crisis. When I took my leave, Charles was ever so tenderly
applying a cold compress to the sufferer's forehead. I have
seldom witnessed such caring as that of this faithful lover.
When I phoned the next day to inquire about James, Charles
said calmly, "He died yesterday, peacefully, several hours
after you left."

I had been visiting Don every week or so for some
months before his cancer of the eye finally spread to vital
organs. I had known him, his young wife, and their three-
year-old daughter for several years. Chemotherapy no longer
held out hope of remission. I thought Don knew he was dying,
although he made no mention of it. I made sure that the prayers and Bible readings I shared with him included references
to death. Marian, his wife, had been told by the doctor that

Don was dying, but neither of them would convey the dreaded news to Don. The real problem was Don's mother. Never was denial more clearly visible. "He's got ten years to go," she responded to the doctor's prognosis. "Give him carrot juice!"

"He knows, I feel sure," Marian confided to me. "Then why don't you let him know that you know, Marian? Why pretend it is not happening? You and Don could share so much better the little time you have together." She did not want to. I respected her wish, but kept gently suggesting to Don that the time was short. I had to respect his right to know.

Finally one morning Don's nurse called me, "He's dying, father. Come quickly." I was the first to arrive. Don's chest was heaving, his breathing rapid. A look of struggling for dear life distorted his face. I sensed his fear, but knew that in his condition he could not voice it. "It's all right, Don," I said. "The Lord is coming for you. There's no need to worry; it won't be hard. One final breath and you will be with Jesus. And Don, you don't have to keep struggling. You may let go when you want to. God doesn't expect you to hold on until the last minute." His breathing slowed. The look of agony left his one good eye.

Marian and two close friends were in the corridor, distraught but wanting to be there at the end. Then the elevator door opened and Don's mother bolted out, wringing her hands. "Is he dead? Is he dead?" "No, Mrs. Walsh, not yet, but the end is near. Please sit down." She took a chair and, with coaxing, seemed to regain some composure. I dared not risk a bedside scene, so I said, "Please, when we go in now, don't make it hard for Don to go." We filed into the bedroom. His mother walked strongly to the head, took Don's hand in hers and said sincerely: "Don, the Lord gave you to me. A better son I could not have had. I give you back to God." Marian took her place and in like words granted him leave. For the next quarter-hour, we took turns talking to him and praying. There were no tears; everyone was calm. Don's breathing slowed.

The next thing I knew, the nurse was removing tubes from Don's nostrils and arms. Annoyed, I was about to order her away. Instead I asked, "Is he dead?"

"Yes," she replied softly. There was no frantic signal for the resuscitation team. No intern was summoned to check eye reflex. Even though everyone in the room had heard the nurse, there were still no tears, no wailing--these came later. We lingered in the room, everyone supporting Don's wife and mother, waking the living.

I was amazed at how easily the end had come. Looking back, I had never been so prepared, so ready with the right word and gesture without having planned them. But I was not surprised. Five months before Don died, I had consulted two charismatics. "I have a problem," I said. "A friend has

cancer. We've been praying for a cure. Twice his wife drove
him to charismatic centers for healing, but there is no sign
of improvement. How am I to know when to stop praying for
a cure and start preparing him for death?" They asked, "At
the charismatic healings, did anyone make an announcement?"
I was not sure what they meant, but I answered, "If anyone
had mentioned a cure, I'm sure his wife would have told me."
"Then it's clear," they said. "There won't be any physical
healing. Prepare your friend for death." I breathed a sigh of
relief, but my relief was short-lived. "Would you like us to
pray over you?" they asked. Chagrined, I felt like saying:
"I'm not sick. I don't need prayers." Instead I said, "Yes."
They took my hands in theirs and we prayed aloud for sev-
eral minutes. "Lord, give courage and guidance to do what
needs to be done" was the tenor of their prayer and mine.
Thereupon they lapsed into deep silence. Thinking the session was over, I sought to retract my hands. They held on.
I waited. After a minute or two, one said simply, "I hear,
'I will give peace.'" The other followed a short time later with
"What comes to me is, 'I will not leave orphans.'"

It was only at the deathbed scene months later I saw
these communications verified to the letter. Never had peace
been more tangible than in that room. The "no orphans" assurance came true during the months of bereavement. Close
friends and relatives wove a web of support around Don's
wife and mother and child. None have wanted for bread or
love. Don's daughter had been spared the sight of her dying
father and his body in the coffin. Only one problem arose.
Now the child lived with fantasies that her father would return. A year's work with a child psychologist dispelled her
fantasy.

These three experiences have taught me several hard-
earned lessons. One, death need not be the bugaboo that our
culture makes of it. Second, knowledge of the stages of
dying defined by psychiatric authors is helpful, indeed indis-
pensable, in Christian ministry to the dying. Third, the
authority of the religious minister sometimes needs to be in-
voked to assure the dying that the effort to stay alive is not
imposed by God and may be terminated by the decision of the
patient. Someone has to tell patients to let go. Fourth, and
most important, the religious faith of the dying and their
support groups can call into play the intervention of God.
It is this dimension of faith that I wish to reflect on. In per-
son-centered therapy, we dare not ignore it. It can be a
valuable ally.

Faith was a sustaining force in the lives of all three
dying persons described here, and in the lives of those who
supported them. For wife, lover, and daughter and son,
faith was the basis for their summoning me, a minister of
religion. Faith led me to respond to their invitations. I felt

drawn to attend, although I had been fearful of death, reluctant to be the bearer of bad news.

For me, the most remarkable thing was experiencing
the faith of the two charismatics who solved my dilemma, then
prayed over me. They believed strongly in a God who heals,
either physically or by imparting peace and strength. Their
faith was matched by Don's, when twice he struggled from
his bed to be driven 200 miles to seek a cure at the hands of
these charismatic healers. For him, faith gave the hope of
improvement. He still had something to live for.

For me, an old saying took on new meaning: the faith
of the healer is what heals. That realization did not come
easy. I am not a devotee of charismatic prayer. Although I
have attended charismatic sessions and approve of the sincer-
ity of the faith they manifest at prayer, I have not felt
drawn to become a member. Witnessing at Don's deathbed the
peace that took over him, his mother, and wife, and seeing
verification of the promise, "I will not leave orphans," my
faith as a professional minister of healing grew by a leap and
a bound.

This is all the more remarkable to me in that I had
been schooled by the church to be wary of self-deception
fraud, and the demonic in religious visions, inspired utter-
ances, and predictions of the future. I had been taught that
the Rules for Exorcism explicitly prohibit performance of the
ritual in the presence of any evidence of a natural (scientific) explanation of the variant behavior. Last, I had been
trained in the spiritual literature of discernment, a body of
writing that seeks to discriminate between authentic religious
experience and that which is illusory or magical.

Finally, I have made the journey from fideism to scientific reductionism. Fideism is a religious error, long rejected
by the church, which spurns cognitive support for doctrine
and trusts blindly in the private inspirations of inner convic-
tions. Scientific reductionism, as we know, holds that behavioral science is the sole source to be consulted for the explanation of religious phenomena. In this regard, I am reminded of the thesis that sociology cannot explain religion.
Science seeks to objectify, to set forth measurable facts, to
analyze phenomena, and to capture their meaning in the form
of sociological conclusions. Religion, on the other hand, is
mainly subjective, internal. Much of its reality escapes the
piercing eye of the scientific investigator. The lessons of
fideism and reductionism I have learned the hard way over a
period of many years. I hope I have now reached Aristotle's
golden mean, a respect for science and religion, two related
disciplines, distinct but mutually beneficial. In the matter at
hand, this means that the medical healer and the spiritual
healer need to be properly respectful of each other's art.
Neither may dispense with the other; each should welcome the

other's participation. Indeed, they should both be members of a support team that succors the dying and sustains the bereaved.

There are further implications of this truth that need to be spelled out. Not being a therapist, I cannot do so alone. I welcome the collaboration of the practitioners of the medical and psychological arts. I offer one observation from the viewpoint of the practitioner of spiritual ministry to the dying.

Spiritual ministry to those who have no faith in personal immortality is quite distinct from ministry to believers. I know of no behavioral study of this category of persons. According to my limited experience, however, denial of death is markedly pronounced among nonbelievers. At death's dread hour, who wants to face personal extinction, a fate that is literally worse than death? To the believer, on the other hand, our ministering can be markedly different. Anger with God and bartering for longer life can be less sharp, the onset of submission more swift with the expectation of life after life. This I found in James's and Harry's deaths. Their will to live was more quickly and readily surrendered. Although, admittedly, it is rare, I surmise that we have all encountered this same phenomenon in the dying who expire in complete peace, with no denial, no anger, no bargaining. Occasionally one meets this in the bereaved. The death of a loved one leaves the pain of separation, but the separation itself is accepted. "Mother was ready for heaven," they say. Or, "It is God's will. Blessed be the Lord!" The answer sometimes is faith of the believer.

11

Pastoral Issues in the Care of Terminal Cancer Patients

Wilbur H. Huguey

Since it is almost impossible to imagine oneself dead, it is not death that cancer patients fear, but the process of dying, with its attendant features of pain and the terrible finality of the separation of human contact. I believe that terminally ill cancer patients tend to meet their own involvement in the death process in accordance with the resources at their command. For most, some of the significant resources will be supportive relationships with doctors, nurses, family, friends, pastor, and church, through which they experience themselves. Should patients lack significant relationships that prove to be genuinely warm, understanding, and accepting, they find themselves estranged, isolated, and without hope, worth, or power in their own eyes.

In order to meet this process adequately, people must not be alone. Emotionally, they need those who will walk understandingly and empathically with them. If isolation and estrangement are greater than the resources mustered to meet them, patients may become bitter, hostile, and rebellious. Denial, then, may be the only resource left to them as they fight vainly against being overwhelmed by what cannot be controlled or understood.

There are wide variations in the understanding of what acceptance of the death process means and what constitutes rejection of it. In my concept, acceptance is defined as the ability of individuals to adjust realistically to a situation, as shown by their ability to verbalize that situation and to exhibit serenity, confidence, quietness, graciousness, personal warmth, composure, relief, curious wonder, matter of factness, or gentle humor. In contrast, I see rejection of that process as tension accompanied by denial tactics such as hostility, forced cheerfulness, fantasies of recovery, depression, sullen fretfulness, whimpering complaint, or preoccupation

with minor symptoms. However, acceptance does not rule out
bursts of anger, realistic but temporary periods of depression, or complaints about realistic deficits in an effort to alter them.

Since death ultimately comes for all of us, we are all,
in this sense, "terminal." I understand terminal situations to
be those in which patients are foreseeably expiring from the
effects of disease. As I use the word "cancer" here, it
should be understood to apply to all malignant neoplasms of
characteristically grave prognosis.

It has been my experience that three sets of relationships make a tremendous impact on patients and may actually
determine, at least in part, their progress in response both
to the disease and the process of dying. These are medical-
patient relationships, family-community-patient relationships,
and, at least for those who express some faith through a relationship with a religious community, pastor-patient relationships.

In 1960, the Indiana Journal of Medicine (the fall,
"Cancer" issue) carried on its cover a full-color picture of
a giant crab superimposed on the outline of a human body.
It seemed to me then and it seems to me now that the crab
is an appropriate symbol of cancer. Cancer is seen as a mon-
strous, devouring, enveloping something, that creeps in all
directions. It seems impervious to the emanations of cobalt,
X-rays, or radium; it seems to defy the efforts of the sur-
geon; and often it seems to be in competition with chemotherapy to inflict the most pain and discomfort. This popular
concept of cancer sees it as a faceless, crawling process that
slowly claws at and devours one's insides. The fact that it is
often almost undetectable from the outside makes it even
more fearful. For most people, it is an entity that is beyond
control, incurable, and often out of reach of even palliative
measures.

For patients, much of the distress is tied directly to
their own identity or concept of themselves as individuals.
Patients' self-image suffers a violent and, in the end, mutila-
ting attack. If acceptance of the disease and approaching
death is to occur to any significant degree, the self-image
must undergo a terrific transformation. The older, precancer
identity must be discarded. Through a process of mourning
and grief, patients must gradually begin to accept an alter-
nate version that approaches more or less closely to reality.
They must begin to see and accept themselves as persons
who have cancer. Instead of regarding death as the remotest
of possibilities, they must begin to look realistically at the
effects of an imminent demise. Only if this is done can they
establish any control or choice.

It is not enough to see this disease through the eyes
of patients alone, for they are not facing it alone. Others

are involved, for good or ill. They can support patients and
be a blessing, or they can make the load even greater. Added to the question of what the disease means to individual
patients must be the question of what the patients and their
disease mean to those who must relate to them. This will inevitably be reflected in both the emotional and the physical
care that patients receive. The relationship between the medical staff and the patient is a primary element of patient care.

It is not my intention to define this relationship, but
to acknowledge its existence as a necessary and unavoidable
part of patient management. In fact, it would probably be
more accurate to call it a medical staff-patient relationship.
However, in the present hierarchical arrangement, the one
who must ultimately make decisions of any magnitude and
assume responsibility for their consequences is the doctor.
Therefore, the doctor is the symbol of all of the various
facets of this broader concept.

With cancer, death is frequently delayed months or
even years. Treatment may be aggressive and aimed to cure,
or it may be less aggressive and aimed at prolonging life.
Treatment may even be simply palliative management of patients during their dying phase. This often requires long
periods of hospitalization. Therefore, medical staff may be
crucial determinants in the emotional experiences of dying
people.

Patients' reactions may vary from obvious fear or de-
grees of anxiety to full flight from their predicament, characterized by avoidance of anything that might remind them of
cancer. This flight may include reluctance to go for help or
treatment. Patients may find it difficult to articulate these
fears because of the feeling that it is wrong to do so or that
it reveals an inability to handle their own problems and,
therefore, indicates weakness. On the other hand, patients
may express anxiety by insistent demands for examinations,
medications, different kind of treatments, or advice. Patients
may identify with other cancer patients they have known and
the symptoms they observed in those patients. They may
then begin a self-fulfilling prophecy by developing those
symptoms and by being certain that the same end will result.
For patients, the disease may represent punishment for real
or imagined wrongdoing. Moreover, many people consider
malignancy to be foul and socially unacceptable. Although
less so now than in former days, some people still consider
cancer contagious, and fear the odors, deformities, excre-
tions, drainages, and incontinences it causes. In short, cancer is not like heart disease, which is considered clean.

Because of the very personal and intimate nature of the
medical staff-patient relationship, it is not always easy to see
the nature of its dynamics at work. Therefore, it is easy for
everyone closely connected to a case to feel that all is going

well when, in reality, it is not going well at all. Then, when hostility does surface, everyone is shocked and surprised and confused, wondering what happened. For this reason, it is well to inspect some of the dynamics that are often at work. One of these is the factor of control.

The whole fabric of modern medical practice is organized around control, specifically the control of disease. The very inability to control terminal cancer is perhaps its most frightening aspect for both staff and patients. In some sense, the very foundation of modern medicine is undermined by this fact. In many ways, society has been brainwashed to look at medicine as a very concrete "science"; it is easy to forget about the "art" of medical practice. When everything else is out of control, there is an especially intense desire to have things nailed down, concrete, and established without exception. Patients do not like to be told that medical science does not know as much as it does not know. It is because of the feelings of helplessness arising out of this loss of control that attempts are so often made to place the blame on something or someone. Physicians and staff members are handy recipients of patients' hostility, not necessarily because they have been neglectful, but because patients' anxiety can only be reduced to manageable proportions by finding some sort of scapegoat.

One means of attempting to regain control is by the use of magical thought. The process seems to be "If I don't think something is true, then it isn't true." Often this is encouraged by staff members to avoid the emotionalism of patients and to make the situation less upsetting to themselves.

Still another means of regaining control is by withholding narcotics. This used to be a very common practice. Although it is much less common now, it still does occur. The modern hospice movement has gone a long way toward changing this practice, which presumably was meant to prevent addiction or the development of tolerance to drugs. When a patient's death is foreseeable, concern over addiction or the development of tolerance has little logical basis, and is most likely a rationalization because control over all else has been lost.

Patients may not only deny having cancer, but their feelings in connection with it, even though they have been informed many times, and quite bluntly, that they do have cancer. In the face of the tremendous amounts of pain and hardship often suffered by terminal cancer patients, one can expect to find waves of anger and irritation directed toward everything and anything connected with the situation. Nevertheless, it is common for patients to cover such emotions, to deny them entirely, or to turn them onto innocent parties, expecially those from whom no retaliation is feared, such as family and friends. Generally speaking, anger at doctors and

nurses (whether justified or not) for not controlling pain or
for inducing pain by diagnostic procedures is often considered unacceptable by both patients and staff, and therefore is
denied.

One subtle method of reinforcing this is the concept of
the "good patient." The patients are "good" if they cooperate
in all things and do not whimper, complain, resist procedures
or medication, and do not disturb or inconvenience the staff.
They are "good" if they accept all things without question
or, if they do question, can be satisfied with simple answers.
The patients are then rewarded by attention, sympathy, encouragement, and even frank admiration of bravery. Infrac-
tions, however, are punished by the withdrawal of these re-
wards. This sets the stage for further tension and disruption
of vital communication between patients and staff.

It has been noted that some patients talk freely and
learn the language, so staff feel that they are clued in and
know what is going on. However, some patients defer or
avoid taking realistic action that might confirm or emphasize
their situation. Delay is one form of denial. Others insist
that their symptoms are caused by factors other than illness
and that things will soon turn for the better. Some patients
refuse to use the term "cancer," preferring instead such
euphemisms as "my condition." One woman of my acquaint-
ance, who had been bedridden for two years and whose leg
and thigh bones had deteriorated to the extent that they had
to be immobilized, still insisted that she was going to get up
and go to church in the near future. Furthermore, she became very angry when she was not reinforced in this asser-
tion.

Some patients project an unnatural lack of concern
about their condition. They say "it doesn't bother me," or
"I have no pain," as if their words magically negate the diagnosis. Others are motivated to desperation tactics, including the use of laetrile, faith healings, and anything that
might promise some relief. Four main types of cancer patients
defer to quacks: the miracle seekers, the uninformed, the
restless, and the straw-graspers. They all have one thing
in common: the necessity of recognizing something totally
unacceptable or at least highly undesirable in themselves, or
finding some way to deny it or destroy it. Unless these patients get help from acceptable sources, it is likely that they
will make unwise decisions and adjustments of a lesser nature
than they are capable of making.

When a surgical procedure is done to remove an organ,
especially a breast, an arm, a leg, or any body part that
patients associate with their appearance or abilities, grief at
this loss is to be expected. However, in our culture, grief
is generally underplayed or disparaged. We tend to admire a
mourner who takes the death of a loved one "well," by which

we mean that the individual avoids an emotional display and gets on with the business of living. We also do this with patients who are attempting to gather the remains of a shattered self-image and see what can be salvaged of themselves. They are often urged to keep a stiff upper lip or to consider how many are worse off than they are. All this is a way of saying to the patients that those near them are afraid they are going to grieve for their losses, and that this would upset them. If they do not suppress their feelings, they will arouse feelings of helplessness, guilt, defeat, and failure among those near them.

In a sense, every death from cancer represents failure: failure of the patient to seek medical help early enough, failure of the physician to act quickly or thoroughly enough, failure of the medical profession to find a cure for all cancers, and even failure of all of society to support the necessary research. Even if both the patient and the physician have done everything possible and know they have done so, they may both feel certain that they did it all a day too late. For patients and, to a lesser degree, for those near them, the every-widening circle of temporary measures represents failure. Each recurrence of signs and symptoms, each new hospitalization is experienced as a new failure. Each time a chemotherapy regimen must be changed, the range of resources becomes narrower. Patients are also subject to an increasing sense of failure, sexual impotence, a tendency toward urinary and fecal incontinence, weakness of muscles and lack of coordination, shortness of breath, and the feeling of becoming virtually infantile. Especially for those who have regarded themselves as being self-reliant, this can be devastating. Some of those around patients may deal with their own feelings of futility by treating the patients like infants, doing everything for them. Thus, the patients become bedfast even earlier than is absolutely necessary, sacrificed to the dispersal of guilt by pampering.

All of these factors, the loss of control, denial, grief, and failure, restrict the flow of real communication between patients and their individual constellations of concerned, significant persons, and thereby isolates patients. The tendency to withhold information, whether justified or not, results in disrupted communication. There is so often so little that physicians can document concretely, either because the variables are so many or because they must wait to see how patients respond to treatment, that they say very little, or put patients off in one way or another. Even when patients strive valiantly to pin them down to specifics, and would be happy to accept a simple "I don't know," it seems very difficult for many oncologists to make that statement. Everyone else around patients can discuss the situation and vent their feelings, but patients aren't supposed to know what is going on. If they suspect, they must keep it to themselves, lest they disturb others. Thus, imagination and fantasies become taboo, since changes in the attitudes or actions of those around them cannot be explained, and therefore are open to various interpretations. At times, everyone, including staff personnel, may tend to avoid patients, even while doing their best to modify the course of the disease.

In terminal cancer, it is not uncommon for patients to be transferred from one service to another or discharged to home and readmitted. This game of "patient football" disrupts their contacts with other patients and with the personnel who serve them. This, in turn, limits the significant relationships open to them. Many times medical personnel and relatives will whisper together beside patients' beds, or will obviously call one another to a hallway to talk in audible tones, under the supposition that the patients do not hear or notice when, in fact, they do hear and notice. It deepens their sense of aloneness and raises the level of their anxiety. Invasions of privacy such as those that occur in teaching hospitals--for example, when a whole group of interns examine a woman's cervix for signs of tumor involvement--take away a patient's sense of personhood and substitute a feeling of being side-show freaks. It is common for patients to feel lost among strange procedures, languages, and equipment. They feel that perhaps they are no more than numbers or cases, whether this is true or not. I vividly remember when one patient was waiting for a brain scan and a staff person shouted down the hall to another, "How many do you have?" Back came the technician's answer, "Two brains and a liver."

Death itself is a form of isolation. Very likely, one of the most prominent concerns for those who are dying is fear of the experience of complete isolation and abandonment by people.

The purpose in considering all these factors is a desire for understanding as an aid in patient management. This was the same goal of the intern who wrote on a patient's chart: "This man has been told he has a reticulum cell sarcoma, a malignant tumor. We assured him of continuing help and support in living with this disease. He now becomes a partner of ours in patient management." Later, when the man was asked what he thought that meant, he replied, "A malignant tumor is a condition that will develop into cancer if you don't take care of yourself." When his pain returned, he began defensive techniques that defeated therapy. Telling him did not, in fact, make him a partner. Neither will this consideration of the problems solve them. I believe that this is a first step in order that these factors may be recognized in actual practice. There is sometimes a temptation for physicians to support these processes by their inner conviction that death and dying cannot be faced realistically by patients (or by physicians). This is not a necessary assumption.

Although use of the term "cancer" is more common now than it was ten years ago, especially among patients and family members, many still prefer less harsh and emotion-laden terms of a more general nature, such as "suspicious," "degenerating," "softening of the bone," "tumor," "neoplasm," "lesion," and others. For the lay person, these terms cloud the issue in ambiguity. Physicians who use them may be saved from having to deal with the varying emotions that are appropriate to the reality of the situation. This may be part of the reason why physicians sometimes disregard patients' questions or consider them as pleas for reassurance unless they become so persistent and so unavoidable that the physicians can find no other out than to answer the patient directly.

Sometimes one sees cancer patients who have been sedated into near, if not complete, insensibility long before their actual demise. Ostensibly, this is done to control pain, to make the patients comfortable. Yet it is hard to shake the feeling that it is also done to protect those who must see to the patients' needs and watch them struggle with impending death.

Hope is seen by nearly all physicians and most medical personnel as a major goal. All of them, in their own ways, communicate the possibility of recovery to the patients. Although it is less rare than in years past, there are still few physicians who are able to sit down with patients and frankly tell them that they will not get better, and then patiently answer their questions about the probable outcome, symptoms to look for, and what can or cannot be done. Some physicians are able to do this, but forget that such information is so traumatic that patients cannot absorb it, and that it must be repeated over and over again. However, because this is time-consuming, many physicians delegate this task to a nurse or someone else down the ladder. These people have seldom received the training to deal with the emotions that such information is going to elicit. Recovery of the physical body is thus the ground for hope, and to admit the certainty of death is to give up hope. Death is then seen as an enemy, and acknowledgment of its presence is seen as capitulation for both the physician and the patient.

Patients are not islands, but people in relationship to other people in whose eyes they see and experience themselves. These others are not limited to the hospital staff, but include friends and family. Someone defined "home" as "the place where when you come, they have to take you in." The light tone of the statement fools no one who has spent much time observing the home care of the chronically ill. The time and the heavy burden of responsibility involved in caring for patients who have long-term or terminal illness places an almost unbearable strain on even the best family relationships. For this very reason, the common assumption that families will automatically undertake posthospital or terminal care, or that if they do, they will be able to meet the emotional needs of patients, is unwarranted. Family members tend to respond to the needs of the patient, according to the meaning of the disease and its residuals for them. For instance, some people may have strong feelings of disgust, revulsion, fear, or shame. Some still fear that cancer is contagious. Fragile relationships are easily shattered, while strong ones that predated the cancer may overcome even strongly negative feelings. Responses of families to cancer patients is probably consistent with their attitudes prior to the discovery of the disease and its terminal nature. Here, also, the same factors of control, denial, grief, failure, and isolation are at work.

If patients are the breadwinners on whom the family has depended, the very roots of their existence may be threatened. When one adds the total emotional context I have described, the failure of almost omnipotent science to find a cure, and the practical considerations involved in the home care of an extremely sick patient, it is not hard to see why many people snap under the strain. Here again, scapegoating is apt to be common. If many family members resort to this tactic, the result will be almost total family disorganization.

Frantic pleas for prayers, insistence on a change of doctors, and resorting to unrecognized methods of treatment may be urgently pushed, not by patients alone, but by anxious members of their families and by their friends. Patients are often inundated by recommendations from well-meaning friends and acquaintances about new treatments, diets, gurus in the field, and which institutions they ought to be involved with for treatment. All of them have heard of new drugs or a new hope of one kind or another, which they press upon the patient until they raise doubts in patients' minds regarding their past decisions.

Family members sometimes become more concerned over a patient's narcotics intake than their doctors are, even to the extent of removing all medicines from the patient's reach and placing them directly in the care of a dominant family member. Narcotics are expensive as well as habit forming. This may be a factor in families' attitudes, but it also gives them something they can do so that control is in some sense restored. If the doctor is not excited over a patient's narcotic intake even after the family has done much complaining, and family members take control on their own, it is difficult to see that they have any other real motivation.

For patients who have terminal cancer, it is especially likely that their final weeks will be spent in a hospital bed, surrounded by paraphernalia, while the staff fights to prolong their lives. These can be very trying times for family. They do not understand what is going on, and the patient's pain and distress arouses helplessness and frustration. If the patient is conscious, they may sense the distress and feel guilty. When staff do not work exclusively with their loved one, they may think it is because "nobody cares." To the staff, these people become a thorn to be avoided whenever possible.

Denial, especially of anger or hostility toward patients, often clouds the clear field of relationships. Patients may fear to express hostility toward the staff for fear of retaliation, but vent it instead on safer objects, such as family members, causing much emotional anguish. It just isn't considered socially proper to react to a sick person as one might to a well person. Consequently, feelings are covered and denied, or retaliation is made in subtle ways. The family seldom denies the fact of the disease, but often denies the feelings involved. Requests "for the patient's benefit" more often mean "for my benefit." Families often say that it would be much better if the patient could be relieved of pain and suffering. Not recognized is the fact that they also would be relieved of the necessity of watching the slow deterioration of someone they love.

Sometimes family and friends speak casually, with little or no show of concern. Almost an aura of indifference settles over the household. One gets the feeling that the real storm will come later. This may reflect a form of denial, in which emotional recognition and pain are put off, or it may be the aftermath of a period of mourning that has proceeded to the point at which death has been accepted and the patient has been written off the records, so that it only remains for the event to catch up with the preparation.

The "image" of the family needs rethinking. Just as individuals have self-images, so do groups like families have an image of what that group is. The family changes from a group of people seeking full, normal fulfillment of their lives, to a group with a cancer victim in their midst. That person is or may become an invalid. This changes the nature and function of the entire group. The patient is seen as changed or changing from a producer to a consumer of family goods and services, from one who shares equal responsibility for family welfare with the others to one who is their responsibility, and who may leave further responsibilities in terms of children, businesses, bills, and financial burdens.

A keen sense of failure bordering on guilt may pervade members of the family. They may feel that they should have recognized the symptoms sooner or, if delay was involved, that the problem could have been avoided if they had only insisted that the patient get help. For husbands and wives, the growing sexual impotence of the sick partner is a major failure that can have far-reaching side effects. The well partner may undergo a kaleidoscopic variety of attitudes and emotions, ranging from early shock, pity, and tenderness to frustration, to a feeling of being an unfortunate victim, and even of being deliberately and maliciously deprived. Hospitals, with their sterile society and their emphasis on individuals as patients, do not have room or are not geared toward family needs, and their philosophy is not oriented in that direction. I have seen a few instances in which ward personnel have arranged to give a husband and wife privacy within a patient's private room, but this is rare. Generally, there is great resistance to having the couple share the same bed and reluctance to engineer a situation in which a romantic interlude could be established. On the other hand, well partners may be so revulsed by surgical changes in the patient or by concepts of the disease that they retreat or are so afraid of hurting the patient that physical contact becomes limited or nonexistent.

Many things work to separate terminally ill patients from their families. The progressive nature of their illness forces them to spend more and more time resting. They are removed almost imperceptibly from the family circle. If patients are not hospitalized, their sickrooms may be far off to one side of the home or upstairs to promote a more restful atmosphere, but their rooms can become prisons. The advantages of home care for the patient can suddenly become disadvantages for the family. Although this is perhaps not a case of "out of sight, out of mind," the family may nonetheless find it less disturbing to have the patient where every moan cannot be heard. They may also find it difficult to cope with paraphernalia and the smells that are often present.

Relatives and friends may suddenly and unwittingly withdraw from the scene long before the patient's death. A common verbalization of both patients and their significant others is "I don't know what to say to them." In some cases, isolation may be actively supported and hostility suppressed by giving praise and attention to patients when they do not complain and withholding praise and attention when their behavior is negative or reveals distress. However, the wearing of a mask, which may thus be considered a virtue, only serves to confuse real feelings.

In later phases, patients may realize the nearness of death and want to talk about it. The slightest mention of this is usually dismissed as impossible or shushed into silence. Patients are reassured over and over again that they are going to be all right, even when all of those involved know that it is not so.

"Patient football" is not a hospital entity alone. Hospitals sometimes discharge patients and send them home "for the good it will do them." Families are also human, and soon find the presence of a dying loved one very upsetting. They then urge the patient to be readmitted to the hospital so that the patient "can be kept comfortable." One woman was shocked

when her husband insisted that she not be given a discharge
to go home. She was absolutely convinced that he did not
want her anymore. After considerable talking, it became clear
that her husband, rather than not wanting her home, was
terrified at the thought. He had encountered trouble in having her admitted this time: if he took her home and something went wrong, what would he do? His fear that he would
not be able to get her back into the hospital had nothing to
do with his love for her.

In my work with oncology patients, several support
groups were established in which patients came together to
share the difficulties that they were having, as well as their
hopes, their dreams, and their fears, and to provide support
for one another in their mutual efforts. One issue that stood
out was that cancer patients tend to feel that anyone who
has not had cancer cannot really understand what they face
or how they feel. In one group that included patients who
had life-threatening diseases other than cancer, difficulties
arose because the cancer patients felt they had less in common with these other patients. It also became clear that no
one can confront cancer patients, zero in on their attitudes,
or reassure them more effectively than another cancer patient can. Until they came to the group, patients commonly believed that they were the only ones to feel as they did. Just
knowing that others were facing the same issues, feeling the
same and reacting similarly seemed to go a long way toward
stabilizing the situation. When one of them could talk about
his feelings, others could share theirs, even though they
had not been able to put them into words beforehand. Still
others were able to sit back and ride on the coattails of
those who were more audacious. Very few in that context
were unable to talk about their cancer, voice some of their
frustrations, share their dreams, provide information and, in
general, just support each other.

If pastors are to support cancer patients in their illness, they must minister not only to the patients and their
feelings, but also to the very source of those feelings. Pastors must also know something of each family's response to
the disease and of the relationship between the patient and
the hospital staff. This is to say that pastors must address
the entire situation from the moment when they become involved with individual patients. They then become involved
as people. What pastors are, what they do and feel, becomes
a part of that total situation. They will not only influence
others, but will be influenced by them and by circumstances.

Cancer, perceived as the great destroyer, promotes an
unconscious attitude of futility in caregivers, and the pastor
is no exception. Perhaps this is one motive behind the prevalent tendency for pastors to see "cheering them up" and
"preparing them to meet their God" as their sole task in re-

lation to cancer patients. Anxiety over the inability to control this disease is manifested by short visits even when the
patients desire longer ones, and even when conversation is
kept to familiar ground, such as the gospel, weather, events
at church, and community gossip. Conversation seldom touch-
es the more personal issues of a patient's feelings. This encourages denial by tacitly urging patients to keep on their
masks and not to disturb their pastors. It endorses primitive
reliance on religion to "make everything all right," sometimes
to the point that patients reject sound medical practice because "God and prayer" are going to make them well. This
is using religion as a shield against reality instead of as an
aid in facing reality.

Because of the nature of the pastoral relationship, it
is not uncommon for pastors to be sought for advice and support by any number of family members on any number of issues, ranging from concern over medical costs and the amount
of narcotics being used to questions about medical procedures,
family tensions, and the behavior of the patient. There is often pressure from family or friends to "see to the spiritual
welfare" of some member of the group. This can become a
frightening load that must be carried on a narrow tightrope.
No wonder some pastors desire not to get too deeply involved.
It is much simpler to concentrate on the patient, visiting often and with much feeling. This usually promotes the gratitude of all concerned: the pastor is so good to the patient,
comes so often, and the visits mean so much. This approach
is less time consuming and means that there is only one person to make demands on the pastor. The fact that all other
matters must take care of themselves is not a pastoral concern anyway--or is it? It is not the fact of the disease that
is denied, but involvement with the family and their predicament. With the pressures of the parish duties, no one will
blame the pastor as long as the patient is not deserted.

When depressed, patients confess a desire to end their
lives and be done with it, or express hostility and frustration, it is not always easy for pastors to refrain from siding
with those who try to convince the patients that these are
not their real feelings. If a pastor accepts these feelings of
the patient, others will look on with suspicion. If the pastor
sides with the rest of the family, the patient is cut off from
any opportunity to deal with negative feelings. Until these
can be considered and accepted, positive feelings will be
buried beneath the weight of the negative ones. Anger and
resentment, universal companions of pain and fear, are not
controlled by logic.

Although ministers may deal with grief more than any
other group of people, grief and its processes are not well
understood. Mention has been made of our cultural approach
to death and grief. If anyone is to aid family members in

realistically reforming the image of their family as a group, or to help patients in working out their own mourning, pastors will usually have to be the ones to do so. To do this, they must understand themselves. They must have thought through their personal attitudes toward death and must be able to recognize their part in the human dialogue.

It seems to me that there is a strange opposition between the calling and faith of pastors and the fear and evasion of death that I find so prevalent. To doctors, death is an enemy. To the patient it means the deprivation of continued contact with family and friends, and may also mean judgment. Although it is possible that death may come as a welcome friend, it usually is, at best, an intruder. To pastors, death ought to hold no fear, but even though they give verbal assent to the belief that death is not without hope, in fact death seems to be represented as hopeless. Pastors tend not to face death realistically or to talk of it openly even when patients provide opportunities to do so. The subject is often evaded by (a) the use of pat answers and doctrinal formulas, such as the question "Are you saved?", (b) by avoiding situations in which discussion of ideas and fears concerning death may arise, (c) by changing the subject, failing to recognize openings, or by responding to lesser themes, and (d) by accepting at face value declarations of readiness for death repeated so often that even a novice ought to wonder whom the patient is trying to convince.

The sad part is that these evasions cut patients off from the opportunity to discuss the very concern that may be greatest to them, their own death and its implications. All others have found it too terrible to face. Now the pastor is unwilling or unable to do so, and the patient is left to face it alone, in a sense isolated even from God.

In accomplishing their work, pastors may be aided or hindered by the images of the pastoral office held by others. These images determine what others expect of ministers. If their expectations are not lived up to or corrected, a pastor is in for trouble and relationships are difficult. For example, our affinity to black and our proximity to the funeral service have not always left a healthy picture in people's minds and may have contributed to the fear sometimes encountered, that if the minister calls, it means you are going to die. Others look on a pastor as a sort of modern witch doctor, whose prayers and Scripture readings are improved versions of tribal chants, guaranteeing magical alteration of the situation if they are repeated loudly and long enough. They will expect the minister to act accordingly.

In the same manner, pastors' images of themselves will guide the way they work. There are several stereotypical ministerial patterns that I have detected among the students and pastors with whom I have come into contact. The first is the Rah-Rah type, whose main purpose is to cheer up the patient. This individual's stock-in-trade is a bright smile, a loud voice, some old jokes, a hearty handshake, and a hasty exit. There is Timid Sam or Samantha, who is scared to death and knows it, and therefore welcomes any excuse not to see a patient. These types feel helpless--if only they could do something--but all they have is the Bible and a few stock prayers. "What is it I am supposed to accomplish?" seems to be their unspoken question. The Medical Experts in Ministerial Garb pass judgment on all treatments, toss around medical jargon, and nod wisely when they get into deep water. Their very presence ought to remove all fear and answer all questions. Then there are The Analysts, whose main interest is in stripping patients of all defensive machinery and getting immediately to the "depth" of things. These people see themselves as "counselors" and feel a need to prove their ability to pierce the patient's psychological armor. There are also The Saviors, interested only in the state of the patient's soul. The first and last item on their agenda is "Are you saved?" If the patient is emotionally upset, it means only that their suspicions were correct: this is a lost soul.

Last, there are The Pastors, Our Heroes, whose main concern is for the person on whom they are calling. They know themselves well enough to be aware of most of their own needs and are constantly aware of their own involvement. They respond in kind to the feelings they perceive in patients, but never to the point of pessimism. Pastors are attentive to surroundings, unspoken conversation, and symbolic terms. They allow patients to proceed at their own pace, in their own direction, speaking of what they want to. Their presence generates concern, and they help in verbalizing the issues that patients are struggling with. Their prayers and Scriptures are discriminately chosen and reflect patient concerns. The confidence that death is not an enemy and that God does care permeates their actions as well as their words.

Theory and practice are necessary elements of patient care and pastoral care. Theory without practice is useless; practice without theory is pointless. One criticism of secular counselors made by pastors is that they have no unifying concepts of the nature of man to guide their work. Religious counselors, on the other hand, have the theory: years of seminary training have carefully indoctrinated them to the religious concepts of man. However, their practice has usually grown haphazardly according to the content of their experience as well as their own innate ability to acquire insights and to align practice with observed response and evaluation. Few pastors are well equipped to do this.

When it comes to practice, most ministers do not feel the guiding hand of their theory. If they did, they would

not be at the loose ends described wherever clergy "let their
hair down." The feelings of helplessness and need to do
something point up the schism between practice and theory.
When doctors enter a sickroom, they have stethoscopes and
prescribed procedures that are understood and accepted by
others. They can do something, even if they feel it is useless. Pastors enter with only their knowledge of the word of
God, their own faith and experience of human nature. They
can only talk, listen, read, or stand silent in the attempt to
understand and help. Others have little concrete understanding of the value of any of these, and tend to assign only a
magical value to them. Feeling this, pastors may be frustrated and, unless they are sure of the connection between
theory and practice, are most apt to evaluate their efforts
in the same way as onlookers do. Our activistic society tends
to evaluate all things in terms of doing rather than being;
when one cannot do, but only be, one is lost. Theory and
practice must be wedded in the laboratory of mutual experience.

Many physicians have written about the doctor-patient
relationship, and some have even included the wider medical
aspects of that relationship. Some social scientists have written about the family-friends-community constellation of relationships. Death and dying courses have become popular in
seminaries, colleges, and community churches. Some authors
have written with insight into the relationship of pastor and
patient. Some work has been done on support-group relationships. However, I know of no effort to put all of these together and to consider them in regard to that major relationship of patients to themselves, focusing on the impact of
those other relationships on that major one.

Whether patients accept or reject their involvement in
the process of dying, this discussion of that process is simply an effort to talk about the relationship of patients to
themselves as they struggle to discard, like an outmoded
garment, their old concepts of self and to forge new ones
more in keeping with the realities of their situations so that
they can find meaning and some measure of peace. I am more
convinced than ever that patients who seem to have everything going for them but who are not surrounded by warm,
supportive, understanding relationships with professionals,
with family and friends, with a religious community, and with
other patients will not, in the long run, make that adjustment. On the other hand, patients whose resources seem to
be extremely limited, but who either have or are able to
form warm, helpful relationships in each of these areas will
go out, maybe not with bands playing, but at least with
quiet, human dignity that says that even this final act has
purpose and meaning.

REFERENCES

Benson, G.A. What to Do When You Are Depressed. Minneapolis: Augsburg Publishing House, 1975.

Benson, H. The Mind-Body Effect: How Behavioral Medicine
Can Show You the Way to Regain Control of Your Own
Health. New York: Simon and Schuster, 1979.

Cassileth, B.R. The Cancer Patient: Social and Medical Aspects of Care. Philadelphia: Lea and Febiger, 1979.

Dawson, J.J. The Cancer Patient. Minneapolis: Augsburg
Publishing House, 1978.

Day, S., ed. Proceedings--Death and Attitudes toward Death:
A Symposium of the Bell Museum of Pathology, The Department of Pathology, University of Minnesota Medical
School. Published by Bell Museum of Pathology and
University of Minnesota Medical School in association
with the Batesville Casket Company, Batesville, Ind.,
1972.

Garfield, C.A., ed. Psychosocial Care of the Dying Patient.
New York: McGraw-Hill, 1979.

Goldberg, J.G., ed. Psychotherapeutic Treatment of Cancer
Patients. New York: Free Press, 1981.

Gray, L. Living with Cancer: How to Help Your Doctors
Help You Back to Health. Pamphlet. Pittsburgh: Life-
line Press, 1978.

Keck, L.R. The Spirit of Synergy: God's Power and You.
Nashville, Tenn.: Abingdon Press, 1978.

Keith, R.L., H.C. Shane, H.B. Coates, and K.D. Devine.
Looking Forward: A Guidebook for the Laryngectomee.
Rochester, Minn.: National Cancer Institute, Mayo
Foundation, 1977.

Kelly, O.E. Make Today Count. New York: Delacorte Press,
1975.

Kopp, S.B. If You Meet the Buddha on the Road, Kill Him!
Palo Alto, Calif.: Science and Behavior Books, 1972.

Kübler-Ross, E. On Death and Dying. New York: Macmillan,
1969.

LeShan, L. 1977. You Can Fight for Your Life: Emotional Factors and the Causation of Cancer. New York: Jove Publications, 1977.

Lynch, J.J. The Broken Heart, the Medical Consequences of Loneliness. New York: Basic Books, 1977.

Nelson, J.B. Rediscovering the Person in Medical Care: Patient, Family, Physician, Nurse, Chaplain, Pastor. Minneapolis: Augsburg Publishing House, 1976.

Oates, W.E. Pastoral Care and Counseling in Grief and Separation. Philadelphia: Fortress Press, 1976.

Rosenbaum, E.H. and I.R. Rosenbaum. A Comprehensive Guide for Cancer Patients and Their Families. Palo Alto, Calif.: Bull Publishing, 1980.

Rubin, J. and C.H. May. Chemotherapy: A Handbook for the Patient and Family. Rochester, Minn.: Mayo Foundation, 1980.

Ruevni, U. Networking Families in Crisis. New York: Human Sciences Press, 1979.

Selye, H. Stress Without Distress. New York: New American Library, 1974.

Simonton, O.C., S. Mathews-Simonton, and J. Creighton. Getting Well Again: A Step by Step Help Guide to Overcoming Cancer for Patients and Their Families. New York: St. Martin's Press, 1978.

Westberg, G.E. Good Grief: A Constructive Approach to the Problem of Loss. Philadelphia: Fortress Press, 1971.

Williams, P.W. When Death Draws Near. Minneapolis: Augsburg Publishing House, 1979.

12

Pastoral Care of the Dying Utilizing Guided Meditation

Joseph P. Dulany

Experience has demonstrated that the value of the approach to pastoral care for cancer patients that has been
used at the Walter Reed Army Medical Center for several
years is contigent on using it with a select group of people.
This group includes adults of Christian persuasion and experience who possess active imaginations, stable personalities,
and the willingness and physical strength to learn and practice meditation. In the setting in which I have worked, these
individuals are frequently separated from their family support
systems.

This approach is grounded in the crisis-counseling theory of Pattison (1976). Primary to his thought is the notion
that the counselor can assist dying individuals in separating
the seemingly overwhelming tasks associated with the dying
process into manageable parts and then assist them in developing coping strategies for meeting the crisis. Pattison suggests that within the three major clinical phases of dying,
key tasks can be identified both for the dying individual and
the counselor.

Commenting on the influence of religion on an individual's response to dying, Pattison (1976) states that "people
whose lives have been imbedded in a religious context will
deal with dying within that religious context" (p. 76).

The basic components of the method are spiritual assessment and spiritual facilitation through guided meditation.
Spiritual assessment of dying individuals begins during the
initial contact with them. The assessment provides a basic
understanding of the way in which individuals are responding to the present crisis, the spiritual resources they bring
to it, and a sense of the way in which the pastor can be
meaningfully involved in resolution of the crisis. The primary
means of gathering information for the spiritual assessment

is listening to the individual's recounting of how they have arrived at this point in their lives. As tedious and difficult as it may be to listen to people's life stories, dying people are best served and the pastoral relationship strengthened by a willingness to hear them out.

In Linn et al. (1979), one of the authors tells of her work with dying nuns and comments on the importance of taking the time to really hear what the dying have to say. She states, "These individuals have never had anyone listen long enough to allow them to finish what they are trying to say" (p. 6). Just listening, no matter how long, is not enough. One must listen with intentionality.

In listening with intentionality, one listens for the metaphors and symbols indicative of the manner in which the individual organizes and shares reality. The person of faith often uses biblical language to describe the concerns and pains associated with living and dying. One should note with equal interest the use or the absence of biblical language in the speech of an acknowledged person of faith. Basic to this approach is a firm conviction that dying individuals, given a caring relationship and ample opportunity, will share the critical and painful issues confronting them. These issues, dealt with one at a time as they surface in pastoral conversation, become the subject material for later work in guided meditation. Once dying individuals have shared their critical issues, particularly those requiring immediate attention, they are gently assisted, through conversation and sharing, to select and claim a Scripture-based incident or text through which to view and work with these issues. Thus, the biblical material becomes the context in which the issue is viewed and worked through in guided meditation. As with the presence or absence of biblical language in their conversation, the manner in which dying individuals approach the actual choice of a Scripture text is an indication of their spiritual and emotional state.

The use of biblical material in pastoral care need not be defended. Its use in a caring relationship has long been advocated by prominent persons in this field. Switzer (1979) reminds us of the special power of the Word as it affects the life situation of the believer. He suggests that Scripture, responsibly used, can not only assist in the clarification of issues and the understanding of vaguely stated questions, but can point the way to the ultimate resolution of issues.

We turn to spiritual facilitation through guided meditation. Once dying individuals' critical issues have been determined and their biblical contexts selected and discussed, they are prepared to experience guided meditation in an attempt to facilitate resolution of the critical issues. In most cases, the individuals will already have been introduced to relaxation exercises (Benson 1976). These exercises, usually considered as premeditative exercises, are taught to most individuals during their first three sessions as a means of helping them deal with the acute anxiety generated by the initial announcement of a terminal prognosis. Relaxation exercises, quickly learned, are highly effective in inducing a sense of peace, calm, and well-being. The side-benefits of relaxation are an increase in physical and emotional energy and a sense of renewed hope. These benefits are welcomed by most dying individuals during these difficult days.

In leading individuals in guided meditation, they are asked to assume the relaxed state. They are then asked to visualize or imagine a particular setting; usually a task is suggested to be accomplished within this setting.

The context of the meditation is predetermined by mutual agreement through prior discussion. It is usually related to biblical material, but may be based on a universal symbol such as a meadow or garden. Individuals are given ample time to experience and assimilate the sensations raised by the guided meditation. After meditation, they are asked to share the imagery and affect elicited by the experience. They are encouraged to bring their own sense of meaning and understanding to the experience. The pastor functions as a caring, sensitive facilitator who allows the individuals to share at whatever level they desire. This time of sharing is a special time, and often assumes a sacred quality. The material generated provides the pastor with the information needed to make plans for the ongoing process.

The responses to the use of guided meditation in work with the dying have varied. For some, this experience becomes a high spiritual moment, often involving a brief sense of self-transcendence. For others it provides insights into the working of their inner being, as well as significant content for future conversations and meditative experiences. For a select few, it is a time of seemingly miraculous resolution of issues: a coming together of faith, emotion, and insight.

This approach, centered on biblically based Christian meditation within a caring pastoral setting (Stahl 1977; Johnson 1974; Kelsey 1976), is more than a method for encouraging emotional adjustment to the process of dying. Although it fully acknowledges and responds to the agony of separation, the pain of extended illness, and a multitude of related issues and concerns, this approach seeks to respond holistically by unashamedly presenting the opportunity for an experience of God's presence through expressions and demonstrations of grace, love, forgiveness, and redemption.

Portions of three sessions with one terminal cancer patient demonstrate the application of this approach at different stages in the pastoral relationship.

S is a Caucasian female, 44 years old. She is the mother of two children, one age 22, the product of an early first marriage, and another three years old, the child of a second marriage. S grew up as a Methodist, and during recent years has been active in a small Baptist church. After she discovered that she had cancer of the breast, she was referred to Walter Reed for further evaluation and treatment. I became aware of her through a call from the oncology nurse, who asked that I see her because of her emotional state. The nurse stated in her referral that this patient was "the worst case of this type of cancer that she had seen in 20 years of nursing." She told me that the doctors expressed little hope that she would be alive two months later.

I saw the patient the next morning. She came into my office openly distressed and tearful. She said, almost as soon as she had sat down: "I just don't know how I am going to handle what's going on. This is too much. I didn't know that I was as far advanced as they say I am." I allowed S to talk, only nodding or giving verbal acknowledgment and encouragement. After several minutes, I suggested that we could work together in an attempt to find some ways she could use to deal with her feelings about what was happening. S said that she needed the help and would appreciate anything I could suggest.

With this opening, I talked briefly about my work with similar patients. I suggested that I could teach S a way to become calm and deal with much of the anxiety she was experiencing. She willingly agreed.

I suggested that she take a comfortable position in her chair, close her eyes if she was comfortable doing so, and simply become quiet in body and mind. I suggested that she trace her breathing, picturing the air coming in her mouth or nose, entering her lungs, going out to the rest of her body, and finally being expelled through her nose or mouth. I suggested that this process was a gift of God to his children. I recalled Genesis 2:7, "And God breathed into man's nostrils the breath of life and man became a living being." I noticed that her breathing was slowing and that her facial expression indicated peace and calm. I left her on her own for several minutes and then called her back, asking that she take several deep breaths, gently open her eyes, and rejoin me in the room. I asked her to tell how this had been for her. "I feel so relieved, so peaceful and calm," she said. "I can't believe it. It was wonderful."

I suggested that she could do this for herself any time she felt anxious and disturbed. I added that if we could work together, I would assist her in learning more about this experience and how it could be helpful to her in future days. She said that she wanted to see me again. We established a meeting time for the next day and she returned to her room.

I worked intently with S during her next two or three hospitalizations. In between, I called her long distance and offered encouragement and support.

The next session I want to relate took place five months after our first session. S was not only still alive, but still vital and active. Our sessions had by now achieved a regular pattern. S came in and usually shared with me the events of the past day. She talked about her treatment, her feelings, her contacts with her family and with other patients in the hospital. Then she usually stopped and either stated her present concern or asked what I suggested we do in this time together. My practice was to shift responsibility to her. In time, she always produced a concern or theme. Her theme this day was the underlying anxiety she was feeling in relation to her disease. I suggested that we work at this issue through meditation.

I asked her to relax and center herself, which she was now able to do immediately upon suggestion. I asked her to picture herself in a safe place. S has been selecting a seascape setting in recent days and did so again. I asked her to visualize the sun bathing her body in its light. I suggested that this light could be God's love and concern meeting the needs of her body. I left her to experience whatever this could be for her. After a few minutes, I called her back and asked her to share her experience. She said:

> This was not altogether a good experience for me. I was lying in the sun . . . it was very bright and I could feel the heat. Then it suddenly became pitch black, and I was confused and scared, really scared. Then streams of light appeared again, but extending upward from me. I felt something leaving me. Something left me.

We sat together in silence, thinking about this experience. I had some notions about what it meant, but I wanted S to think this through for herself. Finally, I asked her, "What did it mean?" She said, "Something left me . . . fears, disease . . . I don't know." I added, "Maybe both. . . ."

S continued to respond to the chemotherapy for the next two months, and then the disease began to gain the advantage. These were difficult days for her. I supported her when she was in the hospital through presence, prayers, sacraments, and proclamation. While she was at home, she meditated with tapes based on Scriptures we had discussed. She also had relaxation tapes with appropriate musical background to use at home. The following session is reported to illustrate how S was responding emotionally during this time when everything seemed to be crashing in on her.

A recurring theme for S during the past few months had been that of dealing with the separation from her three-year-old daughter. In an earlier session, I had used as the basis for discussion and meditation the Scripture related to Jesus' commitment from the cross of his loved ones to one another. S had experienced herself committing her child to significant others in her family and to Christ but, sensing her reluctance in this, I expected that the issue would surface again. During her next hospitalization, this issue did surface, but this time veiled by concern for another child who also was a patient.

S came in and, after the usual period of sharing, stated: "I am concerned about J. She is dying." She told me how she had come to know this child when she met her on the plane coming here. She said: "She was so alive and vital, and now she is near death. She had a serious operation and they don't think she will survive it."

I allowed her to express her feelings, then asked her to think of an applicable Scripture. When she had difficulty thinking of one, I suggested that we think about the time Jesus called the little ones unto Himself and blessed them. After we had talked about this incident, I asked her to go into meditation and visualize Christ accepting the little children as they came to Him for a blessing. I asked her to visualize J and her own daughter with Jesus. After a time of meditation, I asked her how it had been. She replied: "I didn't go along with you. I saw the Lord, but I saw him interceding with the Father. I experienced Him talking about this situation. I don't know what He said, but I know what He was saying was something very important." It was a high spiritual experience for both of us. S was thrilled to think that Christ was involved in her issue.

I have highlighted these sessions to offer a slice of what this approach can do and mean in ministry to the dying. At the time of this writing, although S is still receiving treatment, she remains alive and vital. In this she is a notable exception to the norm. Numerous others who have been assisted through this ministerial approach have "gone to be with the Lord." For many of them, and certainly for S, the quality of remaining life has been greatly enhanced by this kind of ministry to the dying.

The opinion or assertions contained herein are the private views of the author and are not to be construed as official or as reflecting the views of the Department of the Army or the Department of Defense.

REFERENCES

Benson, H. The Relaxation Response, pp. 114–115. New
York: William Morrow, 1976.

Johnson, W. Silent Music: The Science of Meditation. New
York: Harper and Row, 1974.

Kelsey, M.T. The Other Side of Silence. Paramus, N.J.:
Paulist Press, 1976.

Linn, M.J., M. Linn, and D. Linn. Healing the Dying, p. 6.
New York: Paulist Press, 1979.

Pattison, E.M. The Experience of Dying, pp. 76, 318–319.
Englewood Cliffs, N.J.: Prentice Hall, 1976.

Stahl, C. Opening to God, Guided Imagery Meditation on
Scripture. Nashville, Tenn.: The Upper Room, 1977.

Switzer, D.K. Pastor, Preacher, Person, pp. 134–137. Nashville, Tenn.: Abingdon Press, 1979.

13

The Euthanasia Debate and Christian Medical Ethics

Lewis Penhall Bird

For the past two decades, seminars on death and dying have been a part of the academic diet for me as a Christian ethicist. More recently, however, three very personal losses have added new dimensions to this theme. Death, that rude ambassador from the regions beyond, has taken my father, my stepmother, who raised me from the age of five, and my wife's mother.

To recapitulate briefly, my magnificent mother-in-law discovered four years ago that she had breast carcinoma. Surgery was followed by chemotherapy, more surgery, radiation therapy, and that mental paralysis we all know as depression. But through it all, she mercifully suffered little pain, and these physical burdens were balanced with marvelous courage, humor, hope, endurance, faith, and family love. She died the Tuesday before Christmas. When my father-in-law called, his first words to my wife were, "Good news, Carole Ann, Mom's in heaven!"

A few years ago on a summer morning in Florida, my stepmother discovered my father sprawled outside by the flowers next to the garage, mortally wounded by a shotgun blast that had torn through the roof of his mouth and shredded the most fascinating organ of the body, the brain. No terminal illness haunted his last days, but who can know what demons raged in his mind? Ever since 1938, when he lost my mother to cancer--I was four-and-a-half at that time --one reality for my father had been a deeply rooted fear of a similar experience.

Ten days before Thanksgiving, 1981, my stepmother was paralyzed by a stroke while driving home from a Florida shopping mall. Fortunately, my aunt was with her, recognized that something was amiss, and commanded her to pull over to the curb before any serious accident could further

complicate the problem. My stepmother's left side was inca-
pacitated and her speech was considerably impaired. On
Thanksgiving Day, she endured a second, more massive
stroke, which left her with little strength, no speech, and
in a generally unresponsive condition. She survived the
initial episode for just six weeks and one day, dying on the
Tuesday after Christmas.

For me, these were three deeply personal deaths,
providing three new but not terribly brilliant perspectives
on our common enemy. In these circumstances, one learns
much about family dynamics, and about the meaningfulness
and meaninglessness of personal suffering. One also learns
about the quality of medical care in the United States.

Ethicists speak of active euthanasia, passive euthanasia,
antidysthanasia, positive euthanasia, negative euthanasia,
voluntary euthanasia, involuntary euthanasia, eugenic euthanasia, and, in a term introduced by Joseph Fletcher of Situation Ethics fame (1966, 1967), pediatric allocide. Perhaps
the introduction of benemortasia by Dyck (1973) permits a
welcome new perspective; his definition of euthanasia is "a
happy or good death rooted in the Judeo-Christian ethic."

Of interest here are active and passive euthanasia. Few
Christian ethicists are troubled with passive euthanasia, defined as the refusal to employ life-sustaining medical technol-
ogy or drugs to sustain human life further. Medically prolonging human death is a twentieth-century technological in-
vention that Christian ethicists would usually argue against.
Paradoxically, what were viewed as extraordinary means of
delaying death a generation ago have rather quickly become
quite ordinary procedures.

Active euthanasia, however, disturbs most Christian
ethicists. This practice advocates the use of some purposeful
action that terminates life prior to natural death from organic causes. Active euthanasia is often called "mercy killing"
in the face of incurable, perhaps very painful illnesses. After each of three debates in the House of Parliament (1936,
1950, and 1969), English legislators defeated bills advocating
the practice of voluntary active euthanasia. Christian theologians from Augustine to John Calvin, as well as distin-
guished twentieth-century thinkers such as Karl Barth, Die-
trich Bonhoeffer, H. R. Niebuhr, Helmut Thielicke, Bernard
Haring, and Paul Ramsey, have argued against active euthanasia. The eminent Jewish bioethicist, Immanuel Jakovovits,
disapproves as well.

In 1975, when the former president of Union Theological Seminary of New York City, Dr. Henry P. Van Dusen,
and his wife took sleeping pills to terminate their lives in the
face of his stroke and her arthritis, newspaper headlines
read, "Theologian Dies in Suicide Pact" (Philadelphia Evening
Bulletin). Although a philosophical intellectual may have in

mind a well-reasoned ethic of voluntary euthanasia, the lay press and lay people alike perceive only the paradoxical phenomenon of a religious person committing suicide. Curiously, by 1973, 53 percent of Americans polled by Gallup (Reader's Digest) favored active euthanasia "if the patient and his family request it."

Two issues merit review in this brief discussion. The first deals with the control of intractable pain, which so many experience during their illness. LeShan (1964) describes the nightmare of chronic pain in three graphic terms: helplessness, hopelessness, and meaninglessness. One of the major medical innovations of this generation has been the development of the hospice concept. For example, in the palliative-care unit of the Royal Victoria Hospital in Montreal, well over 90 percent of the patients who have intractable cancer pain find comfort and freedom from what Saunders (1967) has called "total pain"; namely, the incredible burden of physical, psychological, spiritual, and social discomfort.

With the memory of my mother's devastating death in 1938 still disturbingly present, I am reminded of Hinton's (1972) lament: "We emerge deserving of little credit; we who are capable of ignoring the conditions which make muted people suffer. The dissatisfied dead cannot noise abroad the negligence they have experienced."

With innumerable U.S. entrepreneurs chasing the health-care dollar, concern for the development of hospice in this country is warranted when such facilities are bastardized by the simple addition of more ancillary personnel to existing nursing staffs. Authentic hospices offer physicians who have been specially trained in the radically different medical procedures of palliative care. Given the difficulty that the elderly ill already experience in finding nursing homes that are run with integrity, as well as the nightmare stories still told by the families of terminally ill patients about the intractable pain these patients endure, hospice care that emerges only as a medical fad or a clinical charade represents the ultimate cruelty to U.S. consumers. However, when legitimate hospice care ministers to the terminally ill, the case for active euthanasia loses most of its advocacy. The sponsor of Great Briton's last euthanasia bill, Lord Raglan, is alleged to have said: "If England were dotted with replicas of St. Christopher's Hospice, there would be no need for a euthanasia bill" (Mount, personal communication).

A second issue worth review in the face of euthanasia proposals is the problem of discovering meaning in suffering. Lutheran ethicist Helmut Thielicke (1964) has been quite candid:

> Euthanasia, which ends the suffering by pre-
> maturely induced death, is contrary to the

meaning of the life of the sufferer. For man,
unlike the animal, is a being who can suffer
ethically. Therefore, there can be a coup de
grace for a dog, but not for man.

A remarkable review of the contradiction in medical circles between treating pain and confronting suffering in the
lives of patients has been presented by Cassell (1982):

> In discussing the matter of suffering with lay
> persons, I learned that they were shocked to
> discover that the problem of suffering was not
> directly addressed in medical education. My
> colleagues of a contemplative nature were sur-
> prised at how little they knew of the problem
> and how little thought they had given it,
> whereas medical students tended to be unsure
> of the relevance of the issue to their work.

The relief of suffering, it would appear, is considered
one of the primary ends of medicine by patients and lay persons, but not by the medical profession. As in the care of
the dying, patients and their friends and families do not
make a distinction between physical and nonphysical sources
of suffering in the same way that doctors do.

> Personal meaning is a fundamental dimension
> of personhood, and there can be no under-
> standing of human illness or suffering without
> taking it into account. . . . Meaning and
> transcendence offer two additional ways by
> which the suffering associated with destruc-
> tion of a part of personhood is ameliorated.
> . . . Transcendence is probably the most
> powerful way in which one is restored to
> wholeness after an injury to personhood.

For clinicians to turn philosophical is always breath-
taking, the more so because their educational processes provide little encouragement or discipline in such endeavors.
Blessed are those physicians who have gone beyond the
cynicism of the residency years and integrated an admirable
philosophy of life with their practice. Twice blessed are
those audiences to whom these clinicians can articulate a perspective that combines informed compassion with good clinical
care.
Those trained in the scientific method know full well
its marvelous facility for discovering physiological truths.
Unfortunately, when confronting life's ultimate questions,
this methodology offers us no help. As Cassell (1982) has

observed, "Reductionalist scientific methods, so successful
in human biology, do not help us to comprehend whole persons."

Discovering meaning in human suffering is no easy
task. When Alsop (1973) was dying of "smoldering leukemia,"
he wrote:

> The most important reason why I felt no panic
> last Saturday was, I think, the strange, uncon-
> scious, indescribable process that I have tried
> to describe in this book--the process of adjust-
> ment whereby one comes to terms with death. A
> dying man needs to die, as a sleepy man needs
> to sleep, and there comes a time when it is
> wrong, as well as useless, to resist.

A year later, when a pastoral friend of William F. Buckley,
Jr. (1975) was dying of Creutzfeld-Jakob disease, he com-
pressed his struggles on paper in this fashion:

> What does the Christian do when he stands over
> the abyss of his own death and the doctors have
> told him that his disease is ravaging his brain
> and that his whole personality may be warped,
> twisted, changed? Then does the Christian have
> any right to self-destruction, especially when
> the Christian knows that the changed personal-
> ity may bring out the horrible beast in himself?
> Well, after 48 hours of self-searching study it
> comes to me that ultimately and finally the
> Christian has to always view life as a gift from
> God, and every precious drop of life was not
> earned but was a grace, lovingly bestowed upon
> the individual by his Creator and so it is not
> his to pick up and smash. And so I find the
> position of suicide untenable, not because I lack
> the courage to blow out my brains but rather
> because of my deep, abiding faith in the Creator
> who put the brain there in the first place. And
> now the result is that I lie here blind on my
> bed and trust in the succeeding, loving power
> of that great Creator who knew and loved me
> before I was fashioned in my mother's womb. But
> I do not think it is wrong to pray for an early
> release from the diseased, ravaged carcass.

> Lovingly given to my congregation and to my
> friends if it seems in good taste.

Wrote Buckley (1975):

It seems to me in very good taste, and I pass it
along, with the good news that at least the final
prayer was answered. The coma began two weeks
later, and on January 21, he died. There had
been no personality change. That, all the dread-
ful powers of Creutzfeld-Jakob couldn't do to
Charles Luckey.

When 43-year-old Orville Kelly was dying of lymphoma,
he founded Make Today Count.* When 17-year-old John
Huneke was dying of bone cancer, he won his Eagle Scout
badge from his hospital bed through the recruitment of more
than 200 new blood-bank donors (1982). These are the success stories. Their opposites haunt us. When my mother-in-
law was in the final stages of her fight with breast cancer,
she emerged one evening from the bedroom, unstable of foot,
half-blind in one eye, her marvelous red hair completely
gone from her scalp. And then this magnificent Christian
woman asked, "Do you mind if I swear?" We all laughed. And
we all knew as well the abiding comfort of the words of the
Psalmist, "Be still, and know that I am God" (Ps. 46:10 RSV).
When intractable pain is well managed--and that is possible more frequently than many hospital staffs understand--
and when legitimate meaning is found in the wide range of
human pathology and trauma, the case for active euthanasia
recedes considerably. Perhaps its appeal is a lingering re-
minder that we are down to the hard cases in pain management, and that many patients are bereft of supportive family
systems and meaningful value systems. Historically and exis-
tentially, helping people discover personal meaning in their
daily lives is what the Christian faith is all about.

---

*The national offices: Make Today Count, P.O. Box 303,
Burlington, Iowa 52601, or call the local office of the American Cancer Society.

REFERENCES

Alsop, S. "Stay of Execution." The Saturday Review of Lit-
    erature/World 1:8 (1973), 23.

Brady, M. "I'll Be Here!" Reader's Digest 120 (721;. May
    1982), 189-194.

Cassell, E.J. "The Nature of Suffering and the Goals of
    Medicine." The New England Journal of Medicine 306:11
    (1982), 639-645.

Dyck, A.J. "An Alternative to the Ethic of Euthanasia." In
    R.H. Williams, ed., To Live and to Die: When, Why,
    and How, p. 102ff. New York: Springer-Verlag, 1973.

Fletcher, J. Situation Ethics: The New Morality. Philadelphia:
    Westminster, 1966.

---. Moral Responsibility: Situation Ethics at Work. Phila-
    delphia: Westminster, 1967.

Hinton, J. Dying, 2nd ed., p. 159. Harmondsworth, England:
    Penguin, 1972.

LeShan, L. "The World of the Patient in Severe Pain of Long
    Duration." Journal of Chronic Diseases 17 (1964), 119.

Mount, B.M., Director of Palliative Care, Royal Victoria
    Hospital, Montreal. Personal communication.

Philadelphia Evening Bulletin, January 29, 1975, p. 11.

---. February 26, 1975, p. 1.

Saunders, C. The Management of Terminal Illness. London:
    Hospital Medical Publications, 1967.

Thielicke, H. The Ethics of Sex, translated by John W.
    Doberstein, p. 266. New York: Harper and Row, 1964.

14

Funeral Rites: Their Impact on Individual, Family, and National Life

Edmond Robillard

From the voiceless lips of the unreplying dead
there comes no word, but in the night of death
hope sees a star and listening love can hear the
rustle of a wing. [Robert Green Ingersoll, American orator, 1833-99.]

When a young man is offered the opportunity to go to
college, he may refuse it, both as a way of showing his
parents that he can resist their will and as a way of proving
to himself that he is master of his own destiny. In truth, by
so doing, he tells himself some big lies. First, he does not
thereby master his destiny, he only makes it different, and
probably worse, than it would have been. Second, he does
not so much prevail over his parents' will as he proves himself to be imposed on by his ill-temper or by jealous friends.

The same thing happens when certain people, by re-
fusing common funeral rites, try to convince themselves that
they will have nothing to do with their own death or the
death of others. Although they fancy that they resist the
will of God or master their own destiny, they only reveal
their inability to assume their human fate as a whole and to
adjust to the conditions of community life. Of course, one
cannot sum up the whole question with such ingenuous and
offhand remarks. Nevertheless, I open my reflections in this
manner as a way of showing that we are not dealing here
with things outside our daily experience and conversation.

There are two things to be considered about death: first,
the way we look at it from inside and feel ready to face it; second, the way it will be looked at and lived by others. In
both ways, our conceptions about death will be shown through
the care we give or do not give to funeral rites. Let us consider, therefore, whether our conceptions are deep enough,

broad enough, and considerate enough to satisfy our admiration for our own selves.

AFRICAN REINCARNATION AS A BASIC EXPERIENCE OF DEATH IN INDIVIDUAL AND COMMUNITY LIFE

Recently a young black student from Africa came to me, complaining that he could not sleep and was in a state of distress: "I believe that I cannot be a Christian anymore." Realizing the seriousness of his case, I had him write a paper on reincarnation, and learned from it a wonderful interpretation of what our own funeral rites should teach us each time we are invited to share in them.

According to the belief of his people, this young student explained, after death people's souls are taken to the Ancestors' Village, where they are judged by the Old Men of the tribe. If it is proved that they have been a shame to their tribe, they are thrown out of the Upper- or Nether-World Village and become demons, roaming throughout the earth as nuisances to everyone. When it is found that they have been good and useful to their fellow men, they are welcomed to the Village of Ancestors, where they enjoy eternal life, joy, and peace. However, there is one peculiarity: in time of need, relatives on earth may pray that dead ones be sent back to them and help them in their distress. If the dead agree, they may be permitted by the Old Men to enter the wombs of pregnant women and be reincarnated.

"That is the reason," said my student, "why I do not want to be a Christian anymore. I want to reincarnate and help my people. But you Christians believe that after death our souls sleep up to the moment of their final resurrection." I do not know how he came to that misunderstanding of the Christian conception of death. "Moreover," he added, "some missionaries, before they baptize us, have us destroy the fetishes of our forefathers, which we keep in our huts. They believe that we adore them, but they are wrong. We adore God only, and believe that He is above everything, we pray to our ancestors because they are the only ones we would dare to bother when we are in trouble."

I have told this story to point out that thousands of years before Christ, human beings devised ideas and beliefs about present and future life while performing long and solemn funeral rites. From the very beginnings of history, humans have devoted care, time, and attention to those rituals, displaying artistic genius at writing poems, singing songs, dancing, building temples, pyramids, and mausoleums, and designing beautiful costumes and dresses, all just for the sake of expressing what death meant to them. Why were they not satisfied to throw dead bodies into ponds, where crocodiles would have taken care of them? Why did the dying not request that their bodies be left to the hyenas along the road when their whole tribe was trying to survive through long and toilsome migrations? What magic or mysterious value had they discovered in burial rites that they even risked their lives to perform them?

I will not give a precise answer to these questions, but repeat what some observers of our modern way of life have already pointed out: that by taking the image of death out of our daily outlook we have brought upon ourselves greater evils than ever came through thinking too much of it. Death has ceased to engross our care and thoughts. Old people now die far away from their families, and children no longer attend the deaths of their brothers and sisters. Death has become unreal to us. In the minds of many, death is like what they see in movies or on television, where those who die on one day come back to life the day after and play new parts in different pictures. This is so true for such people that when they are suddenly brought face to face with real death, the shock is so great that it cannot be assumed, and their minds are thrown out of balance. What then have we gained by reducing the sight of death and by shortening our funeral rites to the utmost? The death of each and every human being--I would even say the death of every living creature--is an event to be matured and digested. If it is not done, death causes a deep and enduring disturbance in human nature. Therefore, if you suppress funeral rites, drop dead bodies into the ground as fast as you can, or burn them in a crematorium, you still do not throw death out of your life, you just prevent that process of maturation and digestion. You hurt yourself and others if they are victims of your haste to get rid of your own or someone else's dead body.

FUNERAL RITES AND HUMAN RELATIONS

We weave social relations for many different reasons: to help our fellow men, to be helped by them, to lord it over them, to enjoy their company, etc. Indeed, the reasons why our modern states and societies hold together are so involved that we seldom dare inquire about them. It is a well-known idea that at the birth of every society there has been a kind of "compact," according to which people have linked themselves together for the purpose of satisfying their common needs. No matter how true or wrong that theory may be, it is certain that the event of death has at times been a reason for people to gather and meet. In the Catholic Mass for the dead, we mention that the departed one "has caused us to forget about our many occupations and trades, and come together as one." But this is only a superficial approach to the

question of our living together. Societies would not live long
on such brittle foundations. Let us then go deeper into that
ground.

Let us go back to my African student and his theory
of reincarnation. There we may realize how profound a link
can be between individuals who share in a certain belief
about death. Being a Roman Catholic, I do not believe in reincarnation. Nevertheless, I would not deny the great part
of truth that can still be derived from that belief. No matter
how different from me my ancestors were, I still carry in my
bones and feelings their features, their bents, and their
likings. Is that not a kind of reincarnation? Childless though
I am, as a priest, I still hope I will be reincarnated some
way in those people who have been influenced by my words,
my deeds, my sound or unsound advice. I should then carry
in my soul deep gratitude for those who made me what I am,
and hope that those whom I have influenced will keep that
feeling of gratitude.

This being said, let us consider our modern way of
life. How are our societies going to hold together if the
image of death is not properly brought forward and proposed
to them? Look at the thousands of displaced people living
among us who have no families, no country ties, no grave-
yards, no memorials. How can we expect these people to develop any kind of family or national spirit? What will keep
those people united? What will make them close to us, and us
close to them?

You have heard of the attachment of Russians to the
"sacred soil" of their country, which kept them faithful to
their emperor in the days of Napoleon, and faithful to Stalin
in the days of Hitler. Let us not say too readily that the
"wages" of fear will easily take the place of that "holy father-
land" spirit in our modern societies. Money divides, and
can be used many ways; fear also divides, and creates more
hatred than faithfulness. Attachment to the dead is less expensive and may produce better results.

Let us understand, therefore, that the preservation or
rejection of funeral rites is not trivial or nonessential in the
life of a nation. Funeral rites not only help people to develop
interest in religion, but to develop an interest in the community life of all of us on earth. They help us to fight
against feelings of loneliness and uselessness, so frequent
in our days, which explain the temptation for individuals to
take refuge in drugs, alcohol, or suicide. Moreover, they
provide a motivation to be as good and useful as possible to
others.

I understand those people who want to be left alone,
both near and after death. They want to break with society
in the same way that society has broken with them. They
hate to think that they might be gazed at in their coffins

under the dim lights of a funeral parlor. They would not
have hypocritical relatives shedding tears on their graves
while making ready to fight for their inheritance. I know!
I know! But how will their own way of acting benefit themselves or their relatives? I understand the considerable suffering that brought them to their present attitude, but would
like them to realize the consequences of their attitude. We do
not allow a father whose daughter has been raped to kill the
rapist, even if he catches him in the act. How can we approve of that other kind of self-justice, which is a violation
of our social compact?

Instead of looking at the worldly side of some funeral
rites, why not look at the teaching they may convey to those
who attend them? What do we know of those who have lived
side by side with us, even though they may never have said
a word to us? Their patience or courage may well have rested on our own. Their decision to go on may have rested on
our own visible determination not to give up! What do I know
of those who want to look once more at my ugly face before
I leave forever? Why should I refuse them that opportunity,
even if it only makes them sure that I am truly dead and
shall no more be a plague or curse to them? We know very
little, sometimes nothing at all, about the odd saints we pray
to in church, and yet it is still good to remember that they
shared with us this earthly life, and were faithful to Christ
and their fellow Christians to the end. Knowing that I have
not destroyed myself, and that I have allowed myself to be
prayed for in the church and cared for by my countrymen
after death may mean more than I suspect, even to those
who are inclined to laugh at superstitions or to scorn the
priestly rabble.

Funeral rites, then, are not only a respectable tradition from the era when it was in good fashion to be taken to
the graveyard in the mourning coach and four or six. It is
truly one of the most ancient legacies from men to men, attesting that there is a difference between a human individual
and a brute beast; attesting the ancient origin and the dura-
bility of faith in the immortality of the soul; attesting that a
human society, like the mystical Body of Christ, is not con-
stituted only of the living, but also of those already dead
and those yet to be born. In that broad context, the care
we take of our own bodies and of the dead bodies of others
is an acknowledgment of the quality and unique value of human life, an asseveration of the fact that we are awakened
to the consciousness of it all.

FUNERAL RITES AND THE DUTIES
OF RELIGIOUS BODIES

Recently, a young priest advised an old lady to buy herself a cheap coffin and to ask that when she died she be taken to the crematorium without delay, even without a funeral Mass. The pretext was her lack of money, but the reason in the mind of the priest was to show a creative spirit by rejecting tradition and to come back to the simplicity of the gospel. I say that there is a long way between the simplicity of the gospel and the simplifications some make of the doctrines of the gospel.

I will not discuss the fact that the Bible tells of some swift obsequies. We remember the old Tobias leaping up from his place at the table and running to the body of a child of Israel lying slain in the street (Tob. 2, 3). Because he had to bury the corpse under the threat of the death penalty, I suppose, Tobias shortened the funeral rites on that occasion. Jesus himself was buried quickly because the Sabbath was to begin with the rising of the first star on Friday evening so that, according to Luke, there was no time for his anointment. Nevertheless, John asserts that Nicodemus brought "a mixture of myrrh and aloes, about a hundred pound weight" to the sepulchre, and "they took the body of Jesus and bound it in linen cloths, with the spices, as the manner of the Jews is to bury" (Luke 23, 53; John 19, 29). I wonder what arguments these actions might provide against funeral rites, so often recommended in the Old Testament and never contradicted in the New?

Surely at times Christian funeral rites have included recollections of former pagan superstitions--the fear, for instance, that the souls of those who were not properly buried might roam through the world and be prevented from reaching the Elysian Fields. However, such beliefs were not common among Jews and Christians, and we see what care they took of their dead, even in times of persecution. We know that a pope and his attending clergy were once killed in Rome because they were caught in the act of performing the regular funeral rites. I recognize that burying the dead with honors and prayers and taking them to a funeral parlor are two different things. Nevertheless, I maintain that there is a difference between both of those procedures and taking the dead directly to a crematorium.

I shall not embark here on a long dissertation on symbolism. However, our most spiritual ideas have to register first in our imagination before they can even reach our mind. Funeral rites are symbolic; take the imaginative symbols away, and you also take away what those symbols convey to the mind. One wonders what price is ascribed to a human life by those who are so eager to get rid of a human body that has been the temple of the Holy Ghost, that has been given to the soul as a dear companion, and that will rise again. What will convey all these ideas to the soul or to our fellow men, if we neglect our funeral rites?

Nothing is truly human that finds no foundation in human nature. Even a religion revealed by God needs to stand on ideas, feelings, and tendencies already present in human nature. Take away those very old and traditional rites concerning death and you also risk taking away the faith, hope, and charity that inspired them. Even faith, hope, and charity, "these three," as Paul would say, so dear to a Christian heart, need a launching ramp before they take us through the stars. That ramp is a natural way of thinking and feeling, expressed through human words, deeds, and symbols.

I do not believe it is out of place to recall the creative spirit and ingenuity displayed by Christianity in adapting the pagan traditions of our forefathers. A pagan rite is never truly removed if it is not integrated into the new belief. Just building alongside is not enough: the old rite must be perfectly substituted by the new one. If this is not achieved, both the pagan and the Christian rites will subsist side by side in the minds of the people, causing a kind of schizophrenia that will sooner or later breed trouble.

Each nation has its own traditions in the matter of funeral rites. Those rites have, through the ages, been the foundation of both the religiousness and the religion of those nations. Take away religiousness and you take away religion as well. A young African who is told to destroy the fetishes of his ancestors may not only stop praying to them, he may stop praying altogether, which would be a deadly blow to his religious feelings. He will not have been made a better Christian, but a skeptic. Christianity will find no launching ramp in his naturally religious soul. The word of God, sown in his heart, will be to him like the seed sown "on the stony ground"; at first it will be received with joy but, having no root, finding there no natural foundation, when tribulation occurs it will be "scorched" and "will wither away."

Funeral rites, therefore, must not be abolished but polished, so that they continue to teach people what they have to be taught today, as they did before. Some individuals have been shocked by and have even been tempted to ridicule what goes on in North American funeral homes, but I believe that by now, even in Europe the way of dealing with the dead has been reconsidered. Exhibiting a dead body that has been protected from decay by embalming does not necessarily conceal the unspeakable horror of death. However, doing so can be a way of reminding viewers that, risen with Christ, our bodies will be made forever beautiful. For mourners to meet in a decent place, surrounded by flowers and sweet music, is not necessarily a profanation, nor is it an obstacle to sincere prayer but may, on the contrary, convey an impression of the peace and rest that awaits us when we are reunited with our dead brothers and sisters. The language of symbols is manifold, and it is up to us to expound them in the best possible way. One thing is sure: I know that some people have been traumatized by the sight of the discomposed features of dear people who have died and, as a consequence, have denied their belief in a God who allows such things to happen. Let our critical sense provide a better understanding of reality, not only of what we would like it to be.

The image of death presented through our funeral parlors should help us renew our relations to God and to other people. The belief in reincarnation is not the sole creed able to establish relationships among the dead, the living, and the yet unborn. We Christians believe in what we call the Communion of the Saints, a Communion and exchange among all those who, from the beginning of the world, have belonged to God. The courage of our Christian martyrs not only inspires us, but also stirs and sustains our courage. Moreover, this affirmation does not come only through saints who have been duly recognized and canonized. Why should not my mother or elder sister care about me now, when they are closer to God, and therefore closer to the universal spring of love and mercy? So is it even with those who helped make this country of ours what it is today. They were not all saints, to be sure, but they did their best, I presume, and may well have been rewarded with the power to help us improve what they started.

I sincerely believe, therefore, that all of this has to be said and explained to the people of all time when they gather on the occasion of death. In these days, when we see family links and national ties becoming looser, we have to look deeper for links and ties that will keep us together. Death can be put to use here. In a world where thousands of individuals are tossed and carried away without having any feeling of belonging anywhere or of being loved or cared for by anybody, it is our duty to bring them back through preaching faith in a kind of Christian reincarnation, wrought through the Communion of Saints, which permits exchanges between the dead and the living.

For all these reasons and many others, I conclude that funeral rites should be of great concern to all members of religious bodies, and most of all to all Catholic ministers. They should at no time abandon them, reduce them, or enter into battle with those whose speciality is to work at the immense task of helping others to make death a deeply personal part of their earthly destiny.

Part III

Loss and Grief

15

The Grief Reaction: A Human Experience

Harold D. Yarrington

During the terminal illness of my stepmother at the time of her final hospitalization, I was able to see her on a weekly basis. She had been informed that she probably had six months to live, and had made her final preparations. She had given the funeral director specific instructions, her Social Security number and her insurance papers, chosen the dress she was to be buried in, and selected a coffin. The family was aware of these actions and approved of them.

After making these preparations, she set her heart and mind on going to heaven and "seeing Jesus." At each of our meetings, she talked of her faith, of Christ as her personal Lord, and her relationship with each member of the family. Her attitude was one of thankfulness to have known each of us. She was able to relate joyous accounts of her relationship to us as our stepmother. Each story or incident related to life in that she would be seeing us again. This was not a good-bye.

This was her pregrief process and we were permitted to be part of the process with her. In addition, we were able to share our faith and love with her in our pregrief. We were able to recount incidents involving our relationships to her. I should note that, for myself, there was a slowing-down process. Some of my remembrances, which were positive and happy, were also a means of denying the approach of death and keeping Mother alive. I also felt some anger, and it came out in irritability with other family members. I masked much of this anger in the many details of helpful acts I could perform for my mother during these last six months. My feelings were ambivalent, swinging from the positive to the negative, from the happy and joyous to the painful realization that she was going to die.

The funeral was held as a celebration of life: her new life in Christ and our new life as we consolidated the family, closing the circle without her and continuing in a new sense of dedication to life. Her life of commitment and dedication, and her faith, which reached out to other people, were spoken of "that she being dead yet speaketh" (Heb. 11:4 AV). Her faith was real and continues to live within our hearts. It is the faith of someone we loved, and who gave totally of herself. We felt a sense of the shortness of life. Therefore, things that needed to be done should be done immediately. I could recognize that this was a postgrief process. Out of this personal experience of the grief process I address some of the areas of concern for clergypersons as they minister to grieving parishioners.

In this account of my pilgrimage in grief, I offer not only my personal perspective, but also some of my instructions to students in clinical pastoral education. Hence, the clinical awareness of human dynamics is highlighted (Blackwood 1942). By using this pastoral clinical approach, we are more able to minister and counsel the grieving. The aware pastor sees the health in the individual as well as the seeds of illness. We are in the front line of preventing mental and emotional breakdown. Therefore, we are aware of the areas of need within individuals and of their need for counseling.

As a clergyman, I have often received calls from people saying that a family member has "passed away." Although these announcements were sometimes expected, they always came as a shock, and my grief was real. I was seldom prepared for the death, either in terms of time or schedule. Even though my stepmother's death was expected, and I had experienced pregrief, I was not prepared. The shock was still there.

My family, like many others who were in the state of basic denial, used veiled terms and double-meaning words when speaking of my stepmother's death. I have found that the easiest route through this difficult circumstance is to deny that the person is dead. The mission of the clergyperson at this point is not to minimize the language barrier, but to help mourners with the reality that the loved one is dead. The church offers mystical and ambiguous terms to soften the blow of death. I feel that this should be permitted, but also that the clergyperson must hold to the point of reality so that the sympathy and grieving of the family will be real.

In ministering to the family, the clergyperson can speak of arrangements for the funeral, helping to choose or notify the funeral director, noting the time and type of the service, special music requested, and the names of those whom the family wishes to participate, such as ushers or pallbearers. All the while, the clergyperson must hold the family to the point of reality: the loved one is dead.

There are many things the pastor can do for the bereaved family. There are things that need to be spoken of, such as which distant relatives should be called. If immediate financial assistance is needed, a church benefit fund may relieve the burden. Officers of the church may assist with transportation and see that meals are brought to elderly members. Help may be needed in understanding insurance coverage. Many people go through crucial experiences and must make painful decisions at this point. This can add to the grief process and cloud issues, so that the grief process is not dealt with properly at the time, or perhaps not dealt with at all.

The funeral offers the opportunity to interpret the meaning of life and salvation, and to find hope in the life, death, and resurrection of Christ. His resurrection is no longer subjective, but a living hope into which the family can enter personally. The funeral also offers the clergy the opportunity to relate to those who are grieving in a meaningful way that they will never forget. They may not recall the words, but the personal ministry will become a part of their lives, a source of strength. The funeral should speak to the life and faith of the deceased. The gifts of ministry and of the Body of Christ should be implemented in a meaningful service. The service should not be used as an end in itself, but as a means of offering the love of Christ and a sense of caring to those in need.

The clergyperson who is aware of the grief process will watch for signs of guilt and anger, although these can be veiled. Guilt and anger will be seen in statements such as, "If only I had been there," "If only I had given him the medication," "If I had kept that doctor's appointment" and "If only I had said or done thus and so." Care should be taken to respond to these remarks appropriately. The natural response would be to rationalize these statements. The person speaking knows that failure to give the final pill or to make the final visit to the hospital was not the reason for the death. This is guilt talking, mixed with anger toward oneself. Anger can come from many directions, and can be centered on a family member, the church, the minister, or even God. The clergyperson should not take this anger personally, nor permit the grieving ones to punish themselves. Nevertheless, guilt and anger will be present. It is necessary to minister to the grieving religiously and spiritually, for their pain involves their total being.

Pastoral care is the quality of feeling with an individual who is suffering. This suffering can be spiritual, physical, emotional, or mental.

Pastoral care is communicating the gospel of God's love through oneself by empathy with those who are grieving. A pastor needs to note certain signs of grief and to interpret them to those who are grieving. This may not be their first experience with death, but each death presents a new and different experience. Confusion is part of the day. Many people will say: "Pastor, I must be going crazy. I don't understand what is going on." Interpret for them that these are feelings of grief, and reassure them that they are not "going crazy." One of these signs is flatness of speech as they relate the details of the death. Some will complain of difficulty in swallowing. They may say that are unable to eat, or that if they do eat, the food feels like a lump in their stomach. They sometimes complain of dryness of the lips, a lump in the throat, slowness of speech, or feelings of depression. They seem to experience inertia, a slowing down, and confusion (Yarrington 1966). Grieving people speak of feeling numb. They leave sentences unfinished. They are unable to sleep, and have deep emotional struggles. They will express fear and emotions that they are not accustomed to feeling. If their symptoms are excessive or last longer than a week or two, they should be urged to see a doctor. Above all, they should not be made to feel guilty about the symptoms they present. They should be comforted with the fact that these symptoms will pass. Through the funeral arrangements, you gave them the opportunity to talk about the deceased. Now, while they are experiencing these physical symptoms, it is important to let them talk about themselves. Encourage them to weep. This is very important for men because in our society "a man is not supposed to cry." They should be encouraged, for "we are to weep with those who weep" (Rom. 12:15 AV). It should be noted that if people react with the opposite of flatness, expressing euphoria, priding themselves on not having cried, or wearing inappropriate clothing, further counseling may be needed. These could be signs of serious trouble.

Encourage the bereaved in their faith in the hope of the resurrection. This will involve assurance about their confession of faith. Help them integrate the Christian message of the death, burial, and resurrection of Christ, from which our faith stems. The realities of faith should also be addressed quite pointedly in the funeral sermon. The sermon should be practical and sharing of personal, loving faith, integrating the message of hope and resurrection as a comfort and assurance. Strengthen that message with the life and faith of the deceased individual. Make a point of showing that the deceased was responsive to others. It is also good to emphasize the individual's own expression of personal faith as shown, perhaps, through a love of the Scripture, a love of the worship service, or whatever that person felt within the Body of Christ. The funeral service should relate to the faith of the deceased as that individual related to life.

When conducting services for those with whom I have not been familiar or those who have not borne a Christian testimony, I bring the Christian message to those who are

present without mentioning the faith of the deceased. A short
eulogy suffices in such instances.

One should emphasize to family members that many past
experiences with the deceased will be remembered with humor
as the days go by. Those lighter incidents will find expression as they come out of the "valley of the shadow of death."
Also mention to family members that anniversaries and holi-
days may be extremely difficult for the first year or two, no
matter how well the grief process has gone. This also depends on their relationship with the deceased and the circumstances surrounding the death.

In many places, it is customary to invite family and
friends to the family home for a repast after the interment.
Use this in your remarks and prayers so that it becomes a
symbolic gesture. Thus, although we have buried our departed, we now close ranks. This meal is a symbol that we
go on living; the nurturing received here marks a new beginning. At this time, also indicate that pleasant memories should
be spoken of with the feeling that the deceased would want it
that way.

The use of Scripture is helpful. The following passages
may be of some help. There are many, and each denomination-
al or funeral service book can assist in the selection of appropriate Scriptures.

> Yea, though I walk through the valley of the
> shadow of death, I will fear no evil; for thou
> art with me; thy rod and thy staff they com-
> fort me [Ps. 23:4].

The strength of this verse speaks of God's presence
even when we are going through a difficult time.

> In my Father's house are many mansions; if it
> were not so, I would have told you. I go to
> prepare a place for you [John 14:2].

This verse speaks of Christ preparing a place for the
believer and His promise of coming again.

> But I would not have you be ignorant, brethren,
> concerning them which are asleep, that ye sorrow
> not, even as others which have no hope [1 Thess.
> 4:13].

> Then we which are alive and remain shall be
> caught up together with thom in the clouds to
> meet the Lord in the air: and so shall we ever
> be with the Lord. Wherefore comfort one an-
> other with these words [1 Thess. 4:17-18].

These verses speak of the hope that as Christ died and rose again, we too shall live in hope. Our comfort in sorrow is in His coming.

First Corinthians 15 speaks of hope, faith, and strength as Paul ministers to the Corinthian church. His message concerns the resurrection of Christ and distinctly relates that promise to life and faith in Christ.

REFERENCES

Blackwood, A.W. The Funeral. Philadelphia: Westminster Press, 1942.

Yarrington, H.D. News Letter. Pastoral seminar, Connecticut Valley Hospital, 1966.

16

Remembering, I Realize—I've Been Where You're Going

Edward J. Mahnke

Twenty-five to 30 times a year the little white frame church opened its doors to receive a coffin and the body of one of its members. The membership gave up time from their fields to pay their respects and join in the funeral service. There was weeping and there was hope. Among these people, used to the cycle of planting and harvesting, death was a part of living. Each Sunday they passed by the graves surrounding the little country church. They checked the flowers and grass plots of their own families.

The country pastor was, by the standard of that day, well educated, but he did not see himself as a scholar. He was loved because he understood his people. When he died, after 45 years of ministry at this parish, the preacher described him as unknown in any place more than five miles from the church, yet known by every person within a five-mile radius of it. He was deeply involved in the ups and downs of the farming community. He suffered when the people grieved and he rejoiced when they were happy.

As a young boy growing up in this setting, I felt I had experienced death frequently and had acquired what I needed for dealing with death and dying. The death of my paternal grandparents was a moving experience. I stood in the living room with the corpse of my grandfather and observed that he really looked dead, so unlike the way he had looked with the twinkle in his eyes and the love in his face when he visited us. But I was not grieving. I believed he had gone to Heaven, and that was better for an old man.

Years later, after seminary, a year of clinical pastoral education, and ten years of pastoral work, I too had experienced the death of patients and had conducted a number of funeral services. I felt confident that my message was positive and hopeful. I, a young pastor, almost indestructible, found death a long way away from me when I was standing next to a corpse.

Then my interest in death and dying was raised by the Kübler-Ross studies. I remember my feeling of smug satisfaction when I was invited to participate in a seminar on death and dying with the entire staff of the cancer unit of the university hospital where I was director of chaplains. The motivation for the seminar came from nurses who were perturbed by their frustration, irritation, and impotence as they daily ministered to and cared for dying patients.

The morning of the seminar, we gathered in a small conference room. The place was packed. People took every available chair, sat on the floor, and stood against the walls. The subject was introduced by the head of the oncology department and, although there was mild tension in the air, in seconds people were describing the frustration and feelings of inadequacy they were experiencing as they dealt with patients who were not being cured. Personal involvement brought pain when death came. The limited opportunities for grieving, inexperience in dealing with grief, and the professional posture were issues that surfaced quickly. These medical people wanted to be good; not overinvolved and paralyzed, but attached to patients and involved with them as they struggled through the days of waning hope.

I listened, my courage and self-confidence growing as each person reported feelings of weakness and helplessness. I could hardly wait for the time for my report. I would tell them that this was really what pastoral care was about, that pastor-chaplains came into these crises with the message of Heaven, which resolves the issue.

Soon it was my turn and I spoke my good news. I knew about death and dying from my childhood experiences. Pupils of the parochial school I attended sang for each funeral. Our teacher was the organist, and because we were not trusted in the schoolroom during his absence, our singing was accepted. That way he could still exercise his supervision over us.

I had grown up in the parsonage. The pastor was a model for involvement with parishioners and a willingness to go with them through the Valley of the Shadow. As his son, I experienced him as an accepting person who was totally nonthreatening. No matter what a person had done, said, or been, through his acceptance he had communicated hope.

Although this model was available to me, I had become a little more detached in my hospital ministries because my parishioners were strangers to me until they arrived at the hospital. I would be acquainted with them for only weeks before I would be asked to officiate at their funerals. I was involved to a limited extent with patients, and in a lesser way with their family members. The text of hope, of Heaven, was available to me, and I could preach a sermon that was positive and hope-filled without really knowing the family members as they carried their loved one to the grave. My message to the grieving was one of eternal hope beyond medical help, which therefore was the solution to the process of death and dying.

"That's the trouble with you preachers!" The nurse turned on me. I can still feel the frustration and see the hurt in her eyes. I knew that she was deeply involved with a parish. I was taken aback and could not understand what had provoked such an outburst. She went on, "You talk about Heaven at a time when people have just begun the process of grieving, and you do not touch them at the point where they are hurting. I am angry when people try to console me with the statement that the person has gone to Heaven when I am hurting because I have lost a patient with whom I had become involved and was close to." Nothing more was contributed that day. I defended my position to myself. First, as I internalized my experience, I said to myself, "She was not in touch with all the hope the church offers her. She was overreacting to the deathbed situation. She was overinvolved with her patients."

Not long afterward, I came upon a head nurse who was quietly crying in a side room. I moved toward her. She told me that one of the patients, a nurse who was dying of cancer, had said, "I always feel better when you are on the floor." The head nurse then added, "But everyone loves Karen so much that they are doing everything for her and there is nothing left for me to do. Everyone who goes in tries to make her more comfortable, and I feel so helpless." It was then that we sat down to talk about the grief she was experiencing because she loved Karen so much. She was a professional peer and a personal friend, and now she could not stop death, could not do anything for Karen. She could only be there. We talked about the termination of every relationship that is begun. None of us can escape it. We realized that whether we marry, have children, or move to another territory, each relationship that is begun must end.

The better, the more satisfying a relationship, the greater the price at the time of its termination. When a relationship has been weak, superficial, or uninteresting, we may look forward to breaking it off. When death ends a relationship with someone with whom we have had a deep and profound experience, we not only learn that the relationship ends, but that the end is very, very final. No longer is it possible to communicate, to do things for each other, to hear the other person respond. And so the loss sets grieving in motion. Grieving allows us, for a little while, to be irresponsible and, if friends and associates will let us, to express our heartfelt loss in our own way.

The most difficult funeral service I have ever conducted was Karen's. I wasn't aware of how deeply I had become involved with Karen and her husband, Bruce. She had asked that I conduct the funeral service, and had outlined its every detail. I began to realize what the nurse in the seminar had confronted me with, as I sat in the pulpit chair waiting for the time when I was to give the homily. I was grieving, but I was to bring comfort, support, and hope to her family, medical team, and friends. The chapel overflowed. Everyone was in tears; people could scarcely speak to each other. We had lost one who had involved herself deeply in each of our lives. I did not want to break down during the service. It would embarrass me not to complete what I had started to do. And I did not want to speak hollow promises of hope that I could not appropriate for myself.

Everyone present could eulogize Karen better than I. In many ways they knew her more intimately than I. Suddenly I was conscious of how, together, we were supporting each other and looking at the model Karen had been for us, in her faith and hope, as she fought to live, as she battled cancer. Her two sons, sitting next to their dad, and the three-year-old daughter he held in his arms drew the grieving hearts and weeping eyes of the congregation. There was impotence: nothing could be done to change or correct what was happening. We were grieving together. I stood in the pulpit, making short sentences of hope for us all to cling to.

Five years before, my father had died. Prior to his death, I had had a particularly strenuous, tension-filled experience. Those were dark days, and I wondered if I would survive without my father, an accepting person who listened, supported, encouraged, and motivated all of us. The morning he had his stroke was a difficult one. My impulse was to fly home and be with him, but that could not happen. I remained in constant contact by telephone, from 400 miles away. I began to distrust the people on the other end, wondering if they were telling white lies.

Some weeks after my father's initial stroke, I was able to be with him. We discussed the possibility of his retirement. I tried to listen, but my grieving was still too important. Eventually, he decided to retire and enjoy the rest of his life. Six years later, he developed prostate cancer and survived surgery. Another four years later, he had a second stroke and was hospitalized. Following the second stroke, he lived for two months. When I saw him he was paralyzed, unable to write or talk, but he communicated by hugging us when we visited.

When he died, he lay in state in the church where he had served as pastor for 45 years. My mother, together with my two sisters and me, stayed in the sanctuary with the coffin when parishioners, pastors, colleagues, and friends came each afternoon and evening for three days. It was then I understood what pastoring and grief are about.

Many clergypersons came, well-meaning personal friends, who put their arms around us and said something fitting, and we were pleased that they had taken the time. There were others who quoted the right Bible passages but seemed uninvolved with us. Sometimes they told us about the deaths they had experienced, and I had trouble listening. I found myself disengaging from them, making ready to receive the next person.

Some came to us at the right place. Those parishioners who had enjoyed my father's ministry for 30 to 45 years felt that he had become part of their families, and on that day they were part of our family. Many of them were speechless, like Job's comforters. Like us, they knew that this death was to be expected, that my father had had a stroke and had cancer, but we were grieving. These callers grieved with us. The first contact was a very simple but profound embrace, clinging to each other and drawing support from each other with tears keeping us mute. When the emotional wave slowed, we were able to share supportive words with each other. One lady said, "Your family is loved." Those experiences in grieving were meaningful. Those people listened with their hearts; they hurt with us, and they wanted to reassure us. They said things that we knew, but with a simplicity of relationship, of feelings, that ministered to us in our grieving. They did not say, nor did they need to say "I understand." Their attitude showed they understood.

What have I learned about pastoring by grieving? I have learned that it is necessary:

1. To live in the world of the bereaved.
2. To listen with our hearts.
3. To avoid imposing values or agenda on the bereaved.
4. To let them share sources of support, love, and anger. God in his greatness accepts even the anger of the bereaved.
5. To understand the great value of physical touch and emotional involvement.
6. To give mourners the freedom to be irresponsible. As long as they are not hurting themselves in their expressions of grief, they should be allowed to pursue them without criticism or judgment.
7. To avoid recalling our own grief experiences. If we have learned from them, it will show in our responses to the bereaved.
8. To realize that grief is not a short-term project. It requires at least the cycle of a year. Each anniversary must be passed until the first anniversary of death comes.
9. To not fear our uneasiness as we approach grieving people.

10. To respond to grieving, rather than to structure a protective film that makes us impervious to the experience of those who grieve. We must feel, listen, and remind them that they are loved at a time when everything seems so terribly dark and lost and out of control.
11. To accommodate requests from the bereaved for the reading of favorite Scripture passages or the recitation of certain prayers. Such observances can have great meaning to the bereaved. We must not think we will be heard for our many words.
12. To allow mourners to deal with grief and loss in their own way.

Eventually rational behavior moves into emotional reaction, and life goes on as glimpses of daylight appear at the end of the tunnel.

17

Pastoral Care of a Congregation and Pastor

Perry H. Biddle

At 1 A.M. on the morning of Thursday, March 22, 1979, there was a fire at the First Presbyterian Church in Old Hickory, Tennessee. Neighbors behind the church building discovered the fire and awakened my family--we live next door to the church. As flames leaped from the roof of the building and firemen attempted to control the fire, but to no avail, a sense of anger and shock moved through the crowd that had gathered. Our house is only about 15 feet from the church building, so my family began removing valuable items from the house in case the fire should spread.

Immediately, I called several leaders of the congregation to let them know about the fire. Some of them came to view the destruction. Others who live at a distance stayed awake the rest of the night thinking about the implications that the fire would have for the congregation. There was a general state of shock and disbelief among those who saw it happening. For several weeks after the fire, I found myself denying that it had happened. I avoided looking at the ruins when I was near the burned-out building. The church secretary, who occasionally came by the ruins, had the same experience of shock and disbelief.

The emotional shock was so traumatic for me that I became physically ill on the morning after the fire. I was scheduled to teach a class on funerals and grief at Vanderbilt Divinity School in Nashville, and I managed to go. I began by sharing the loss that had occurred with the class of divinity students and explained that I might have to excuse myself at any moment to go to the restroom because of the grief reaction I was experiencing. This sharing of my intense shock and pain became part of my own grief therapy as I "owned" my feelings with a group of caring persons.

That same morning, members of the congregation gathered to assess the damage and to begin salvaging items from the church. This act was therapeutic. As individuals walked in among the charred ruins, they were shocked into realizing the devastation wrought by the fire. Young people as well as adults were involved in this, and it made a real impact on all of them.

After the initial shock, many parishioners expressed strong emotions. Some wept privately in their homes; others expressed to one another their anger, frustration, and disappointment. As pastor of this congregation of 160 persons, I called a neighboring minister to arrange for church services the following Sunday so that members could share their feelings. We had a "townhall meeting" of the congregation following the worship service at the Old Hickory United Methodist Church in order to air our feelings. One woman expressed her fear that I might leave the congregation because of the fire. Many others may have felt this fear but were unable to express it. I had no intention of leaving the congregation in crisis and made this clear at that time.

At that meeting just three days after the fire, parishioners expressed a strong feeling that the church must be rebuilt "just like it was." This same feeling is found among those who suffer the death of a loved one and in their grief, attempt to restore the deceased to life by keeping that person's room just as it was and by setting a place at the dinner table. This strong feeling of wanting to recapture the lost object was widely shared by members of the congregation.

As we expressed our anger over the senseless burning of the sanctuary and fellowship hall, which caused a loss of $300,000, we sought to place the blame on someone or something. In spite of several inspections by the state fire marshal's office, the cause of the fire was never definitely determined. The fire seems to have begun in the area of the gas-heating system in the basement, leading to some suspicion that it was caused by a defect in the heating system. However, a week earlier, during the Wednesday prayer meeting, another church a block down the street received a phone call in which the anonymous caller said, "The Presbyterian Church is on fire." The fire marshal discounted this as a crank call. We sought to discover why anyone might have wanted to burn the church. Many felt that if we could fix the blame for the fire, it would enable us to express our emotions toward the guilty party or parties. However, this was never possible.

The evening after the fire, the church officers met in my home to discuss plans for the future and to share our feelings. We also spent time in prayer, asking God's guidance for the congregation. One elder, a scientist at the DuPont plant nearly, gave thanks to God that there had been no north wind that night, which would have fanned the flames and caused them to destroy a whole section of the village of

1,400 houses. This expression of trust and gratitude toward God and his providential care of property and life was one of the more significant expressions in the early days after the fire.

One of the emotions strongly felt was devastation and defeat. We began to issue a newsletter every other Monday. The newsletter, which we named "The Phoenix," expressed our hope that, like the legendary bird, the church would rise again from the ashes, although we did not know where or how that would happen. We learned that many people shared our grief and sense of loss, and would rally to our support. They generously gave financial gifts as well as love and encouragement.

We attempted to channel our feelings into constructive activity rather than self-pity. There was, as usual, some self-pity, but for the most part members turned to the future and what could be done to rebuild. The afternoon after the fire, I met with one of the leaders of the congregation and we made plans for a planning committee of officers and members to do a thorough study of the church, the community, and the surrounding areas, and then to recommend to the congregation where and how to rebuild the church. This committee met regularly, and prayed and shared together. It employed two professionals who specialized in helping churches to relocate. Outside assistance was very valuable during the entire process.

During the weeks and months after the fire, we expressed our feelings to one another in the church service, during my pastoral visits to members' homes, and through talking with one another. I felt the support of the church members, other clergy, and friends during this period. I did not feel depressed or lonely. To the contrary, I was driven by the demands made on me for leadership to deny some of my anger and loneliness. (I did experience several months of depression after the church had been rebuilt.)

During our recovery from the fire, I was called out of the community to represent our denomination as a commissioner at our General Assembly meeting and was involved in several out-of-town meetings. I felt pressure to get away from it all from time to time. I was not aware that any of the church members were aware of what I was experiencing, since they were caught up in their own grief. (This often happens to a husband and wife when a child dies. Neither is able to comfort the other adequately because they feel their own grief so deeply. The likelihood of divorce among such couples is much higher than normal.)

Few churches have fire-insurance policies, but we were blessed with one that called for full replacement of the building. The officers of the church had taken out a new policy just six months before the fire, and the limit of the policy was $300,000, the exact amount of the damage to the building. This enabled the congregation to recover emotionally and financially without being crushed by a huge debt.

In spite of this security from the insurance company, there were still moments when we all felt panicky. We were in a crisis and did not know how it would work out. There were times when some of us would have liked to escape from it all, but the loss wouldn't go away. We had to deal with it. The congregation decided, by a vote of 54 to 40, to rebuild the church in its old location, rejecting the recommendation of the planning committee to relocate six miles away in a new housing area. Since I, as the minister, was associated with the planning committee and supported its recommendation, some of those who were leading the movement to rebuild in the present location felt hostility and resentment toward me. This was a difficult time for a number of people who ordinarily were rather passive "saints" of the church, and some of them also expressed hostility about my having been out of town on several occasions.

In addition to the insurance that covered the rebuilding of the church facilities, my office library was covered by my household insurance. My books were declared a total loss from smoke and heat damage. Several friends and churches helped to replace my library. These acts of support were very healing and helpful as I faced my loss.

We were able to return to our usual activities of church school, worship, covered-dish suppers, and other programs immediately after the fire, through the generosity of the nearby United Methodist Church. Our church offices were relocated in two of their vacant basement rooms. I found it very supportive to be in their building, since we have secretarial help only two days a week, but there was someone in the Methodist church every day. The two ministers of the church, who were friends of mine, were very affirming and supportive. They and many of their church members gave me valuable pastoral care. Later we moved to a junior high school cafeteria, where we had more space and could hold services at the usual time of 11 A.M. We found that hope gradually began to come through as we saw the building being rebuilt and as we worked together to make a new beginning.

Finally, a year and a day after the fire, the time came to move into our rebuilt facilities. We were able to buy and install a used pipe organ to replace our electric organ. A few minor changes were made, but otherwise the facilities had been rebuilt "just like they were" before the fire. Our lovely stained-glass windows in a contemporary style had been replaced, and the pews and furnishings matched the originals as closely as possible. We were even able to return to our facilities free of debt and with a sizable amount of money left over in a bank account.

Several weeks after moving back in, we dedicated the rebuilt facilities. This was a great celebration as we affirmed, once again, the reality of our life as a congregation in our own building. An overflow crowd of friends, as well as members, came to help us celebrate on a Sunday afternoon. Part of the congregation watched the services on closed-circuit television in the basement.

In this paper, I have attempted to trace the stages of grief of a congregation and pastor after the loss of their church by fire, showing how this loss parallels the loss of loved ones to death. I have been able to deal with the grief caused by the fire and to help my congregation deal with it through an understanding of the normal symptoms of grief reaction. I submit this description of one grief reaction, trusting that it will enable other persons and groups to cope more effectively as they respond to losses in their lives.

18

Judaism and Pastoral Care: Dying, Death, and Bereavement

Audrey K. Gordon

Skillful pastoral counseling in Judaism is often a matter of personality and a mature philosophy of life that is based on experience rather than on specific skills learned during rabbinical training. Many rabbis specialize in unrelated academic fields and are not particularly adept in the interpersonal situations that arise from the crisis of dying and bereavement. What follows is an attempt to clarify ideas and events in the Jewish tradition that might offer the Jewish pastoral counselor some insight and guidelines when calling upon Judaism to offer comfort and hope to those who are dying and to bereaved families.

It seems to me especially important to discuss the diverse ideas about death presented in the Bible, since Judaism itself does not readily provide theological clarity on the subject. In addition, I provide some guidelines for counseling dying and bereaved Jews that are consistent with Jewish tradition and secular wisdom, and a look at the dynamics of the customs surrounding the funeral and mourning process. This may offer a better understanding of how these traditions can be used for healthy grieving.

The Bible portrays the concepts of death and dying in various ways. The etiological question of why death exists is answered by the Adamic myth of sin through disobedience in the Garden of Eden, with death as one of the punishments decreed by God: "The man has become like one of us knowing good and evil; what if he now reaches out his hand and takes fruit from the tree of life also, eats it and lives forever" (Gen. 3:22 NEB). The form the dead take is poetic justice as well as reality: "You shall gain your bread by the sweat of your brow until you return to the ground; for from it you were taken. Dust, you are, to dust you shall return" (Gen. 3:19 NEB). From this citation comes the Jewish tradition

of using only organic materials (wooden coffin or linen
shroud, for example) to enclose the corpse for burial. This
is done to ensure the speediest decomposition of the body to
its natural "dust" state. Consequently, it is prohibited to
use any materials (metal coffins, preservative fluids, or her-
metically sealed vaults) that might preserve the body from
natural disintegration. Death, the writer of Genesis seems to
say, is divinely ordained, final and total; it is part of the
natural process of growth and decay.

The Psalmist and Deuteronomic writers report another
view of death. Among many ancient peoples, death was seen
as a weakening of the energy level (nefesh) necessary to sustain life. If you were too weak to live, you went down to
Sheol where you existed in a faded, listless dimension that
still required minimum sustenance.

It was a custom in ancient Mesopotamia for hollow tubes
to be placed at the head of the grave. The family of the deceased poured foodstuffs into this tube in order to sustain
the deceased in the netherworld. This concept of death as
diminished energy but not as loss of consciousness is found
in First Samuel, twenty-eighth chapter, where Saul calls up
Samuel from Sheol to inquire whether or not God is on his
side in the battle against the Philistines:

> The woman answered, "I see a ghostly form
> coming up from earth." "What is it like?" he
> asked; she answered, "Like an old man coming
> up, wrapped in a cloak." Then Saul knew it
> was Samuel. . . . Samuel said to Saul, "Why
> have you disturbed me and brought me up."

Ancient customs still echo in our traditions of visiting
grave sites when we become engaged or married, and consult-
ing the dead when making important decisions, as portrayed
in Fiddler on the Roof.

The Psalmist presents a picture of Sheol as a place
from which God is absent. Only the living can praise God.
"None talk of thee among the dead; Who praises thee in
Sheol?" (6:4-5). The rhetorical questions are to be answered
negatively: "Dost thou work wonders for the dead? Shall
their company rise up and praise thee? Will they speak of
thy faithful love in the grave of thy sure help in the place
of Destruction?" (Ps. 38:10-12).

The Psalmist's argument for restoration hinges on the
rationale that God requires praise from man and cannot be
praised too abundantly. Through references such as those in
Psalms, Proverbs, and Ecclesiastes, we gather a picture of
the realm of death as a cheerless, stagnant place to which
all must inevitably go. It is necessary that all go there, for
if the corpse is not securely interred in the ground that is

the doorway to the land of the dead, then the spirit will haunt the family. This idea is paralleled in Greek and Roman religion, which requires descendants to feed their ancestors in their tombs lest they turn from gods into malevolent demons.

From this configuration of ideas concerning the importance of remembrance, we can relate to the Jewish traditions concerning the duties of the onen to suspend the performance of ritual laws until the dead are buried and observance of the memorial Yahrzeit remembrance, which may be a modern vestige of surrogate ritual for the offering of sustenance at the grave site.

Koheleth shares the Psalmist's view of Sheol as a deprivation of God's presence, but with less angst. For him, death is the obliteration of consciousness and life, under any circumstance, is preferable to death:

> But for a man who is counted among the living
> there is still hope: remember, a live dog is
> better than a dead lion. True, the living know
> that they will die; but the dead know nothing.
> There are no more rewards for them; they are
> utterly forgotten. For them love, hate, ambition,
> all are now over. Never again will they have
> any part in what is done here under the sun
> [Eccles. 9:4-6].

In the Book of Daniel, a note of judgment is added to this bodily resurrection: ". . . many of those who sleep in the dust of the earth will wake, some to everlasting life and some to the reproach of eternal abhorrence" (Dan. 12:2).

The theology of bodily resurrection plays an important role in Jewish laws concerning treatment of the body. In Orthodox and Conservative Judaism, there is belief in a personal Messiah who will raise the dead in the World-To-Come (Olam Ha-Ba). Because the physical self will rise, it is necessary to preserve the body and all its parts (including parts previously amputated) in the grave. Autopsy, which involves removal of body parts for examination, is forbidden unless mandated by civil law, as is embalming, which involves removal of the blood. The purpose of these prohibitions is to safeguard the intactness of the body at the time of its resurrection.

This issue of intactness prohibits organ donations in many cases but, with the development of heart transplants, Halachah was interpreted to allow the donation of a critical organ in order to save a specific life. Specificity is the key to permitting an organ donation. There must be a particular person who needs the organ in order to live. Jewish law preeminently maintains the importance of saving a life to the ex-

clusion of any other legal requirement. However, this orthodox interpretation does not permit the donation of kidneys,
eyes, bones, and other body parts to organ banks, which
distribute them to recipients who are not known at the time
of the donation. Jewish laws that prohibit cremation and the
scattering or mutilation of body parts stem from the concept
of bodily resurrection. However, the custom of burying Jews
with sticks in their hands so that they can dig themselves
out of the grave when the Messiah comes is now rarely observed.

Of what value is all this to Jewish pastoral counselors?
By presenting different biblical views of death, it is possible
for counselors to ascertain whether a dying or grieving person's view of death is of biblical origin. The increased di-
versity of the biblical positions allows counselors to offer
more helpful solutions to questions about death or life after
death than perhaps was previously possible. Not everyone
wants to believe that life exists after death. For some, the
notion of extinction, or "dust to dust," is just as comforting
as bodily resurrection is to others. The Book of Ecclesiastes
has a very modern ring in its espousal of living as fully as
you can, "for already God has accepted what you have done"
(Eccles. 9:7). Offering God's acceptance of the life already
lived is a way of reinforcing God's continuing approval of the
person and of extending the assurance that whatever lies
after this life will not include punitive judgment. These
thoughts and such others that emphatic counselors can offer
can go a long way toward easing the fears of abandonment
and anxieties about wasted life that many dying people experience. Perhaps it needs to be said that pastoral counselors should not espouse points of theology without being sure
of their own positions. It is not necessary for them to believe them all (indeed, that is impossible) in order to suggest
alternative answers that may suit another person's needs.

The Bible reflects the life and customs of ancient times
--the Halachah reflects the wisdom of rabbis and sages in
meeting needs with interpretations that permitted the survival of the Jewish community over the centuries. How, in
the twenty-first century, will we respond to these beliefs
and prescriptions from the past?

Although Freudian psychology is a fairly recent historical phenomenon, many of the laws and customs, and much of
the folk wisdom of Judaism are rooted in sound psychological
understanding. The Jewish rituals of dying, death, and bereavement have much evidence of such understanding.

The Halachah commands us not to abandon the dying
either during their illness or their final hours. Psychologically, the greatest fears of death are not usually of death
itself, but of the process of dying. We fear abandonment,
loneliness, suffering, and separation. Death means a loss of

relationships. Judaism enjoins us not to desert those who are dying for even one moment until they have reached the security of the grave and the attention of God. We are commanded to alleviate that which we fear most. Studies indicate that loneliness potentiates the experience of pain, and that the presence of a caring community diminishes suffering.

Much has been written in the last decade about Kübler-Ross's stage-theory of dying (1969). This theory was welcomed with relief at the prospect that perhaps there was a way of understanding what dying people go through, and that with this understanding, caring persons could help to meet the needs of the afflicted. Kübler-Ross's theory was a valuable step forward in an area where few steps had been taken. Since then, closer scrutiny of dying people has forced us to make some modifications of that theory.

Although the Kübler-Ross model of stages--denial and isolation, anger, bargaining, reactive and preparatory depression, and acceptance--accurately describes the feelings of terminally ill people, it is not correct to suppose that different people experience all of these feelings or that they necessarily do so in the order initially outlined. Kübler-Ross herself has repudiated the notion that the order in which these feelings occur is invariant. People do not neatly go from denial to anger to bargaining and so on. What we have learned is that people die as they have lived--some angry, some accepting, some denying, and that many people experience combinations of these feelings over a period of time. The coping mechanisms of a lifetime and the individual personality are very much in evidence in this, the final challenge and stress of life.

In what ways can pastoral counselors be of benefit? What information is needed to provide comfort, and what stance is the most honest and supportive? First, pastoral care-givers must know something about each person to whom they give counsel. If that seems obvious, we should remember that many Jews have only a formal relationship with a synagogue and know little of "their rabbi" other than from High Holy Day services. This is clearly not the rabbis' fault, but the expectation exists that rabbis will be able to move intimately into the family circle to offer perfect comfort and counseling because it is their job to do so.

Questions that the pastoral care-giver must keep in mind as a checklist are:

1. How has this person coped with other losses?
2. Were there healthy ways this person coped with loss?
3. What does death mean to this person right now?
4. Can I strengthen this person's ability to face what lies ahead by focusing on these coping mechanisms or developing new ones?

5. What other people are available in this person's support system? What can they realistically do?
6. Although I may be operating in an official role as rabbi, does this person really want to talk to me about the most intimate issues of death and dying? Will I be offended if he or she does not?

Each person has a different fear and special understanding of the meaning of dying and death. We must listen to hear their fears, not our own, and we must not hasten to reassure them with platitudes, theological or otherwise. People who are dying have unbelievable fortitude and control over their own lives and dying, if they can be made aware of this power. They are not infantile, passive, or piteous unless we encourage them to be. They deserve honesty in all things (including diagnosis and prognosis), compassion, and our help so that they can live out the rest of their lives as adult human beings in as much control of their bodies as is medically possible. They need to know that the person "keeping company" with them recognizes and respects them as autonomous adults with minds and souls intact. Although their bodies may be deteriorating, it is to these minds and souls that we must speak with love and dignity. To do otherwise is inhumane.

Pastoral care-givers can, by example, show families how to interact with their ailing family members. The counselor demonstrates to the family that open, honest communication is not destructive but helpful, that sharing of feelings and tears can be appropriate, and that the ingrained dynamic of withholding bad news from loved ones and not speaking about negative happenings is not to be practiced in this situation. At a time of crisis in family life, it is possible for family members to strengthen their ties to each other. However, any student of family dynamics knows that in time of trouble, a dysfunctional family does not function better-- indeed, it functions worse. Many people would like to see their dying family member through this time with love and compassion, but the reality may be that too much has gone on before to allow psychic wounds to heal completely. We must not fault family members when this is the situation, nor insist that maintaining a united front is the only way for a family to function.

It is not humanly possible to predict the exact hour of death. The requirement for the Jewish community to be present at all times relieves the family of guilt feelings they might have if they were not with the dying person constantly. It also fulfills the religious commandment of recitation of the Sh'ma at the moment before death, either by the dying person or a member of the community. Confession of sins (vidui) prior to death is a rite of passage from one stage of life to

another (from this life to life with God). This eases the heart
and mind of its burdens and can give the dying person permission to "let go" when life can no longer be lived. At this
point, the rabbi's tasks with the dying person are to communicate God's forgiveness and acceptance through confession
and recitation of the final ritual, leading to utterance of the
Sh'ma.

When the loss that death represents overwhelms us,
many times we wish to die also. We not only identify with the
dead, but can also see death as an escape from the pain of
grief and the reality of life without the loved one. Here the
duties of the onen function as an important psychological de-
terrent. The definition of onen describes the status of the
mourner (father, mother, sister, brother, husband, wife,
son, or daughter) before the burial has taken place. It is
the duty of the onen to make whatever arrangements are necessary for the funeral, suspending all other religious obliga-
tions in order to perform these tasks. Mourning (here dis-
tinguished as attention to one's own grief and the receiving
of ritual comfort given by the Jewish community) may not
properly begin until after the funeral. This activity of the
onen serves to reaffirm to the bereaved that they are alive,
have responsibilities to fulfill, and may not sink into the
numbness and oblivion of depression and self-negation. At a
time when we might wish most strongly to die in order to be
with our dead loved one, the tradition insists on life and
familial responsibility.

The grief process is painful. Sometimes, in kindness,
friends or relatives attempt to shield the mourning family
members from making personal decisions about the conduct of
the funeral service or the disposal of the body. However, as
psychologically painful as it may be, it is more therapeutic
for mourners to be involved directly in these decisions than
to experience the funeral service and burial as a personally
decisionless ritual. Direct involvement with funeral arrangements fosters a sense of continuing care for the deceased,
as well as recognition of the finality of death, which is so
necessary for healthy grieving. Sedation for the mourners is
not advised. I remember one well-meaning family who, when
their father died, sedated their elderly mother for the funeral and shivah week. When she emerged from her semicomatose
state ten days later, her first questions were "What happened?" and "Where is my husband?" She then had to face
her painful feelings alone, without the comfort of community
and rituals.

Much that has been written about funeral directors in
past years has left the impression that they are motivated by
financial profit and either too callous or ignorant of the Jewish traditions of burial. My experience with Jewish funeral
directors has shown this to be basically untrue. We, as con-

sumers, are largely responsible for the direction that the Jewish funeral has taken because we have abdicated our right to make decisions and to express our wishes in keeping with the traditions. In the absence of guidance from family members, funeral directors follow the most efficient or most socially accepted procedures for the community they serve. A popular misconception should be corrected: embalming is not required by any law (state, city, or federal) unless the person has died of an exotic disease such as typhoid or cholera that is potentially dangerous to others. Jewish tradition spares us from the U.S. way of putting the dead on display.

The lack of artifice and the simplicity of the traditional Jewish funeral serves other good psychological purposes. The reality of the death is not denied if the dead are not cosmeticized to appear as if they are "sleeping." The ritual washing of the body (taharah) by the Chevrah Kadishah is a loving act by the Jewish community for one of its numbers, reaffirming that even in death the Jew is safe from strangers. The natural state in which the body must be kept speaks to and reassures our deepest psychic fears of mutilation, which we all share in some measure. The shroud (tachrich), the rabbis said, reminds us of our equality before God--that we appear before God with no external coverings to distinguish us as to status or wealth, only that we are Jews. The immediacy of the burial not only provides therapeutic activity for the mourners, but also shifts the focus to the mourners as quickly as possible so that they may begin grieving and return to living fully that much sooner.

The demand for simplicity in the Jewish burial averts the misuse of guilt feelings, which are another common psychological dynamic of grieving. When people we love die, we feel guilty because they are dead and we are not; because we are angry at them for dying and feel guilt over that anger; because we remember times when we did not behave lovingly toward the dead; because their death is a relief to us; or because we did not love them and we think we should have. Frequently a way of defending against these feelings of guilt and anger is to lavish funds on expensive funeral arrangements to convince the world (and ourselves) of our loving feelings for the dead. While assuaging guilt and anger in this way may work for the moment, recognition of these feelings when they are especially troublesome and working them through in counseling is extremely important in order to avoid later psychosomatic damage. Extensive studies corroborate theories that unresolved grief can cause later mental malfunction as well as heart attacks, colitis, ulcers, and other physical problems, and even death.

Jewish rituals furnish clues to the inner dynamics of the grief process. The tearing of clothes, Keriah, or its more abbreviated form, the tearing of a black ribbon, signi-

fies the internal anguish at the tearing away of a loved one.
The fabric of life has been torn by the death. Modern society tends to trivialize the rituals and symbols of death in an
effort to deny the death and its most obvious implications.

When we do not wear outward symbols of mourning, we
participate in death-denial by not permitting society to comfort us or respond to us as vulnerable persons in need of
care, as we are. Symbols of mourning, such as the torn ribbon, make us as wounded persons. They signify the need
for a helping response from the community. When we deny
our vulnerability, we deny the fact of the death and the reality of our pain. When garments are torn, they may be mended after the shivah, but never so completely that the scar of
the tear is not visible. The separation is not mended; the
loved one has still been torn away. Nevertheless, the hurt
and pain will heal, leaving a scar.

The funeral service itself contains several spurs to the
open expression of grief. The purpose of the eulogy (ches-
ped) is, through praise of the dead, to make the mourner
aware of the magnitude of the loss suffered and thereby
bring tears. El Malay Rachamim, heard many times before,
for the first time is heard with the name of the beloved. The
recitation of the Kaddish at the cemetery with the mourners
standing at the grave site reemphasizes the reality of the
death and reaffirms the bonds among community members,
one with another, as they collectively remember and re-
experience their own times of mourning with the newly bereaved. The Kaddish, extolling the greatness and inscrutabil-
ity of God's ways, sanctions the outpouring of anguish by
controlling it within a prayer praising God at a time when we
are most likely to want to curse God. It protects us from
our own desire to vilify God, an action we might later regret.

The work of the burial itself is to be done, at least in
part, by the mourners. This is the final act of "putting to
rest" that again helps mourners confirm the reality of the
death and fulfills the mitzvah of safe burial for loved ones.
Artifice here also should be shunned. The raw earth is real-
ity--"dust to dust," the tradition demands. A word of warning: the managers of a few cemeteries are so crass and un-
feeling that they have a bulldozer visible and waiting at the
grave site. The funeral director may be asked in advance
for hand burial in the Jewish tradition if the weather permits.
If a bulldozer must be used to finish the task, at least that
can be done after the mourners have left the cemetery
grounds.

After the burial, the mourners return to the house of
shivah to find the "Meal of Recuperation" (seudat havra'ah)
prepared for them. Hard-boiled eggs, with their rounded
shape, are a traditional symbol of the fullness and completeness of life. They also signify the ancient sacrifice in the

Jerusalem Temple, as well as the implicit fertility of new life. The egg represents life, just as the meal provided by the caring community carries the message of life to the mourners. The act of eating also carries other messages. Mourners are not permitted to ignore their physical needs or abuse their health--they must go on living even though at that moment they may wish to be dead. The community says, "We are here to feed you even though your loved one is no longer here to answer your needs. You are not alone. We can help care for you now when you feel weak." This first mandatory meal is a resocializing experience, reinstating the mourner within the realm of the living and within the patterns of health.

The most important task of the week of shivah that now begins is telling the "story of the death" repeatedly, so that the death is verified and placed into the perspective of the family's history. Only when the family can assimilate and cope with the details and events surrounding the death will they be able to talk of the meaning of the life of the person who is now dead. When we can remember the lives of the dead, their significance for our lives, their feelings for us and ours for them, then their positive contributions to us as persons continues into our future lives. It is when we cannot (or will not) remember the dead that their lives truly cease. It is important to note that within significant emotional relationships there are always negative as well as positive feelings. Recalling these negative aspects of the dead and our feelings about them is a therapeutic part of the healing process of mourning. When we overlook this aspect of our relationship with the deceased and elevate them in memory to unwarranted sainthood, we again deny the reality of the lives that have been lived and the loss that has been experienced.

Many people experience discomfort when visiting the newly bereaved. This can arise out of a sense of inadequacy, a feeling of being unable to comfort the mourners in the face of the severity of their loss. Visits to the bereaved can be anxiety-producing confrontations with our own mortality, leading to a subconscious feeling of relief that we are not in the same situation (a universal human response). The wisdom of the Jewish tradition rescues the uncomfortable comforter by decreeing that the mourner makes the conversational overtures and the visitor listens. In this way, the comforter comforts by sharing what the mourner wants to share and by not intruding into areas where the mourner does not wish to go. Silence is very often a warm, participatory, caring experience when it is understood that no conversational burdens are necessary. The custom of bringing sweet foodstuffs to the house of mourning symbolizes the Jewish belief that life is sweet and worth living. The injunction not to work during shivah recognizes the need to pay attention to oneself, and not to be distracted from the grieving.

Judaism recognizes that there are different levels and stages of grief, and organizes the requisite year of mourning into four parts: the first three days of deep grief within the seven days of shivah and abstention from normal social functioning, 30 days of gradual reabsorption (sheloshim) into the community, and 11 months of remembrance and recovery. The mourner is slowly drawn back from the numbing isolation of loss toward responsibility and concern for the living, so that at the conclusion of the year of mourning the loss has been felt, worked through, and accepted, although not forgotten. The Jewish custom of lighting a memorial candle on the anniversary of a death (Yahrzeit) structures a circumscribed time in which the feelings of grief may be permitted to reemerge for expression and examination. Feelings of continuing grief thus are sanctioned and limited within a religiously controlled framework, reinforcing the Jewish view that joy in life is God's wish for us and sorrow, although unavoidable, should not be the pervasive tone of our life experience.

Too often, the modern pace of living seeks to shorten or abrogate ritual. Mourning rituals provide the wayside markers for open and appropriate expressions of grief. They say, "Now it's all right to cry"; they identify, "Here is someone who's hurting"; they comfort with "God is in control of this situation even if I am not." When we deny rituals, we cheat ourselves of time-tested and sanctioned avenues for the healthy expression of intense emotions that arise when a death occurs. A death causes a painful, bleeding, internal wound for the bereaved; participation in meaningful rituals advances the healing process.

The role of the pastoral counselor or clergy as a facilitator with the bereaved is fairly straightforward. Here is where the rituals and beliefs of Judaism are most comforting, especially when their origin has been explained in a context that makes sense to the listener. The rabbi can explain the Jewish traditions of the funeral process, pointing out why, in some households, water is used to wash one's hands after returning from the cemetery, what the duties of an onen are, and so forth. When a family is able to distinguish law, custom, and superstition (as with the covering of mirrors), then they can understand and personalize their ritual experience--they can feel more in control. The rabbi can be most helpful in encouraging a family to make the funeral service very special by including eulogies from friends and relatives, favorite Bible verses, and poetry.

The rabbi also makes sure that services are conducted in the home during shivah. There is often a complaint from young adults that the shivah house has a "party" atmosphere that seems out of place. I attribute this to the natural wish to deny the death, questions about personal mortality, and confusion about what is appropriate behavior at such a time, factors cited earlier. By showing others how to listen to the mourners and by explaining the meaning of the Jewish traditions, the rabbi may help lessen the anxiety of visitors and diffuse the party atmosphere.

After the tumult of shivah has ceased, there is a tendency for people to leave the mourners alone, as if they need private time to recuperate from all that has happened. This is partly true--they do need some time for reflection--but what is not stressed is that this recuperation is best when supportive people are very much involved in the mourner's lives. The continuing presence of the rabbi, synagogue community, and friends is needed to alleviate the desolation and isolation which mourners feel immediately after the shivah period.

Abnormal grieving may not be immediately apparent. It is beyond the scope of this work to detail all the symptoms of normal and abnormal grief. If, however, abnormal grief reactions are observed after six months or so, the rabbi, depending on the depth of his psychological training, should suggest therapy and, if necessary, make a referral.

Pastoral care throughout the year of mourning is shared by the entire synagogue. Do mourners in the congregation have someone to spend Passover with? Would they like someone as a companion going to and from services? Do they need someone to look in and be sure there is food, medication, and conversation? Imparting the feeling that "you are not alone in your time of trouble" is the most important idea that we, as Jews, can communicate to our bereaved, and the tradition of doing mitzvot for others transmits this feeling.

We have had much experience with sorrow in our history. One of the lessons we must not forget is that sharing sorrow lightens its burden. From my own experience in leading bereavement groups, I can suggest that synagogues should form ongoing support groups to help their bereaved members. In addition, a special cadre of volunteers should be designated who will be available to provide funeral advice, food, and services, and to visit during the time of bereavement.

The wisdom of the centuries-old Jewish traditions about death and dying is consistent with our psychological knowledge about healthy grieving and the humane treatment of the dying person. Judaism survives as a way of life because it has built within it the answers to constantly emerging social problems and religious questions. We must look into the future in an attempt to see what social forces and concerns might necessitate creative religious thinking and liturgical and ritual refreshment to meet the needs and identity of Jews of the future:

1. The women's movement is a fact of modern life. Equal-rights movements within Judaism are struggling: they have gained basic recognition from one another, official recognition from Reform Jewish organizations, half-hearted ambivalence from Conservative citadels, and silence from Orthodox bastions. Specifically concerning the rituals surrounding death and dying, Jewish women must be allowed to recite the Kaddish for a loved one, to conduct and be part of a minyan, to be official pallbearers, and to participate fully in all the religious rituals of mourning so that their grief can be permitted its fullest dimension and focus.

2. Funeral costs can be taxing to all but the most affluent families. A return to the simplicity and dignity of the Jewish funeral can include the use of a pall, a cloth covering, to drape over the coffin so that the plainest, least expensive coffins may be chosen. This pall, which might be adorned with significant Jewish symbols, could be the property of either the synagogue or the funeral director. If the funeral service were returned to the province and grounds of the synagogue, the need for building elaborate funeral establishments, with their high overhead costs, would also decrease. Some synagogues, because of lack of space or theological prescription, will still require the use of funeral establishments, as will those families who are unaffiliated with a specific synagogue. The funeral director provides important and necessary services to the Jewish community. It is the material purchases adjunct to these services that must be reevaluated and limited, not the services themselves. Most funeral directors will say (and rightly) that they provide what people demand. Therefore, when we change our notions of what constitutes an appropriate Jewish funeral, the funeral industry will change to meet our needs. Reinstating the Jewish traditions of the equality of all persons in dress, the simplicity of coffin and burial, and the natural dignified treatment of the body will restore the funeral to its appropriate place in Jewish ritual rather than its often slavish imitation of the U.S. culture at large.

3. Ecological concerns and family mobility will continue to be important issues in the future. Although Jewish tradition calls for burial in the earth, this may become increasingly difficult. Fewer Jews buy grave sites in advance because fewer maintain permanent residences throughout their lives. Cremation may become the preferred method of body disposal in the future because an increasing population calls for a different use of available land. We cannot, as Jews, ignore this reality and the need for an alternative funeral choice. Those Jews who now choose to be cremated (Reform Judaism permits cremation) find themselves without appropriate rituals to bridge the gap between the funeral service and the Shivah.

The finality of the graveside service and mourners' inner expectation, based on past experiences, that the burial is where
the finality of the death is made evident are lost. Mourners
are left psychologically adrift, not able to go from Ritual A
to Ritual C unless Ritual B follows in its due course. The
comfort of structure, of course, is that we can follow it automatically without additional effort. What is needed in Judaism
is the development of liturgy and ritual for cremation. At
what point should the Kaddish be said when the family arrives
at the crematorium with the body? What prayers can be re-
cited when the urn of ashes is delivered to them to be interred in a columbarium or buried under a family marker?
What practices must be discouraged as being un-Jewish (display of the ashes, the use of ostentatious urns, and so
forth)? These and other questions have not been adequately
answered, so that Jews who now turn to cremation find themselves religious outcasts, forced to adapt to Christian or secular styles.

4. With the advance of medical technologies, questions
about the prolongation of life and the "right to die" have become commonplace. We must have Jewish answers to these
questions to preserve the quality of life as we understand it.
The concern for the preservation of health for "life" is at the
bedrock of most Jewish law. Judaism has always permitted
passive euthanasia. When Rabbi Judah the Prince was lingering and suffering in his dying, his servant-woman went outside to his disciples, who were praying for his life, and threw
a jar of water from the roof into their midst so that they
would cease their prayers for him. They did so, and he died,
ending his suffering. Sefer Chasidim (Nos. 315-318, Frankfurt
Edition), commenting on the statement in Ecclesiastes that
"There is a time to live and a time to die," says, "If a man
is dying, we do not pray too hard that his soul return and
that he revive from the coma; he can at best live only a few
days and in those days will endure great suffering; so this
is 'a time to die.'"

When the path to death is clear, the Jew may not inter-
fere with the death. There are clear-cut Jewish prohibitions
against active euthanasia (intervention in the dying process
to hasten death), although there has been much discussion of
it. Physicians may not do anything to hasten death, but they
can remove the causes of the delay of death (Moses Isserles
in the Shulchan Aruch and others). Some Jewish groups have
given support to the concept of the "living will" as being
within the Jewish ethical framework. The living will requests
that there be no prolongation of life if suffering and death
are inevitable, and that narcotics that may hasten death be
administered to alleviate pain. Some have interpreted this use
of narcotics as active euthanasia. As a people who know and
condemn suffering, how can we abdicate our responsibilities

to those who suffer and look to us for relief? We must have more discussion and reach a firm modern Jewish position on this problem.

These are some thoughts on death, dying, and bereavement within Judaism. Other issues, such as organ donation, have not yet been considered, but must be. The purpose in exploring sensitive issues is to enable us to live happier and more meaningful lives within a community of support. Death and loss are inevitable; happiness and growth are not. What is life without the boundary of death to give it value? Whether death ends our existence as finite beings is not a question we can answer with certain knowledge. It is an answer of faith. But the fact of death can make us value even more that which we love in life. The original choice to be alive was not ours, but until the "season" of our dying, life, itself the gift, must be chosen as a way of reaffirming God's purposefulness in our creation. And when death comes, it is as the extinguishing of a candle, whether its flame is flickering or burning brightly at the end. Wither goes the smoke and the warmth?

19

Christian Witness and the Terminally Ill

William C. Mays

The proliferation and overabundance of materials on
death and dying have created difficulties for some of us. We
can find little enthusiasm for most new books on death and
little interest in yet another journal article, tape, or autobio-
graphy by a terminally ill patient; we are not much motivated
to attend new seminars on death. Perhaps it is that after
being exposed to a certain amount in this field, we begin to
meet the same things in a rehashed or disguised form over
and over again. The law of diminishing returns sets in. At
this point, what more can be said about the inner experiences and emotional needs of dying patients than has been
by Feifel, Bowers, Jackson, Kübler-Ross, Glaser, Strauss,
Weisman, Hackett, Nighswonger, Mills, Butler, LeShan, and
Pattison? An exception to this question may be the subject
chosen as the focus of this paper. Many authorities deal with
counseling the dying in terms of such matters as "death with
dignity," "acceptance," and "the discovery of meaning," but
few struggle with the particular Christian content and dimensions of this experience. Although several speak of supportive pastoral ministry to dying church members, few want to
venture into the area of Christian witness to non-Christian,
terminally ill patients.

Our reluctance to deal with Christian witness is under-
standable. Many of us come from traditions in which "witness"
is equated with a strong-armed evangelism that intrusively
asks, "Are you saved?" "Do you know Jesus as your personal Savior?" "Where will you spend eternity?" and so on. This
has seemed so distasteful to most of us that we have neglect-
ed or rejected any form of personal Christian witness. But,
to use a tired expression, perhaps in the process "we have
thrown out the baby with the bath water." It is the contention of this paper that we, as Christian ministers and layper-

sons, have a clear responsibility for some kind of witness to
dying patients who are without religious commitments.

The relevance of this subject depends on one's eschatology. Is there really a dimension of existence beyond our
present one that we may validly call "eternal life"? If there
is, will it make any final difference if one is a professing
Christian or not? Will not the love and grace of God, after
all, include everyone? Is it, in the final analysis, important
that a dying person confess Christ? This writer's answers to
these questions have led him to struggle with Christian witness and the terminally ill.

The approach is idiographic. The writer's ministry to
one terminal patient will be presented and some tentative
guidelines deduced.

CASE ILLUSTRATION

Jed White was a 53-year-old white male with a wife and
two children. His daughter was grown, married, and lived in
another community. Jed's 12-year-old son attended grammar
school. The family home was in a town about 60 miles from
Nashville. When Jed's lung cancer was diagnosed, he was
initially given a series of radiation treatments, which had little positive effect. Later, as a palliative measure, he was
given chemotherapy. Jed was given positive support and almost constant care by his wife and an older sister. The sister tended to dominate the setting when she was present.

In the beginning, my ministry was one of friendly, low-
keyed presence. I would sit with him to listen, reflect, and
shoot the breeze, but I took care never to push. I discovered that Jed was not a church member or professing Christian, but that his wife, sister, and children belonged to a
local church. Jed and I became friends. According to Jed, he
and his wife and sister looked forward to my visits. After
his family initiated it, Jed welcomed prayer at the end of
each visit.

Some weeks went by in this manner, and Jed slowly
lost ground. He never mentioned God or the church. When I
sought an opportunity to discuss my concern with Jed's wife,
she voiced similar feelings, and we agreed that I should take
a more aggressive approach. The following day I found Jed
alone, and after the usual kind of "passing the time of day,"
I wondered aloud if Jed had been thinking any about God
and how God might be related to him in his illness. Jed admitted that he had been doing a lot of thinking about this.
I sought to clarify what Jed's thinking had been. It became
clear that he wanted "to get things right" between himself
and God. He already had some vague, ill-defined ideas of repentance and faith. I tried to explain and amplify these mat-

ters and then suggested that Jed take some time to think about our conversation.

A day or two later, I visited Jed and again found him alone. And again, after some introductory chitchat, I raised the religious issue. Yes, Jed had had time to think, and had decided that he wanted to make a commitment to Christ. I patiently led him in a prayer of confession and acceptance. Jed was elated, and immediately spoke of his desire for baptism. In consultation with his family, this was arranged for a couple of days later. After his baptism, Jed was received into the membership of the local United Methodist Chruch. In the days that followed, I took Jed some rather simple religious literature to read and encouraged his questions. He seemed satisfied and basically at peace until, one morning, he died very suddenly.

Parenthetically, Jed never reached Kübler-Ross's goal of acceptance. He seemed to retain some remnants of denial and bargaining until the end. It is fair to wonder if his conversion was a part of his bargaining. It may have been, but I nevertheless evaluate his conversion as authentic.

THE INITIAL APPROACH: IMPLICIT OR EXPLICIT

Any pastoral call presents Christian ministers with an initial decision about their professional role. Should their approach be implicit or explicit? Is it enough to be introduced or known as a pastor or chaplain, or must one quote Scripture and speak the language of Zion to establish one's identity clearly? I contend that with the unchurched, the pastor's professional role should usually be implicit. Oates (1958) speaks of keeping a permissive, relaxed relationship and warns that "the bible often reduces permissiveness, creates tension and introduces elements of threat into [the] pastoral context." Being explicit about one's role can have the same result of reducing permissiveness, creating tension, and introducing elements of threat. My initial approach to Jed White was to let him know who I am. If religion in general or the Christian faith in particular were to be discussed, he would bring it up. Prayer with him began only at his family's initiative.

PASTORAL PATIENCE

The second element in the ministry to Jed White was what Southard (1981) calls "pastoral patience." For mo, "pastoral patience" includes two elements: interested, concerned care and alert, but relaxed, waiting.

I visited with Jed two to three times each week, trying to make my calls when he was not pushed and could spend some time with me. Jed's wife and sister were usually there, and although I tried to be sensitive to their needs, my intentional focus was on Jed. And I waited. I waited for Jed to express some religious concern, to raise some religious issues, or to express a need for meaning and purpose in his life. Southard (1981) reminds us that "we must look patiently and perceptively for the teachable moment when a person has 'ears to hear.'" With Jed, such a moment was never obvious.

One might ask why I did not pick up on Jed's interest in prayer. Was this not the entrance I sought? Couldn't I have said: "Jed, you seem to want prayer. I wonder if this says something about your need for God?" Perhaps I should have, but it never felt right. My intuition was to wait. It has been my experience with others that waiting is usually enough. They bring up the subject; they lower a drawbridge over the moat and invite us across. Waiting for them to do so can be an act of faith. Pastors and chaplains believe that God's spirit is active in the life of the other person. It is the Holy Spirit that convinces and mediates grace and faith. Southard (1981) writes: "The 'pastoral' evangelist is one who recognizes conversion as a process which must be consummated in God's time (kairos) rather than a convenient hour (chronos)."

INITIATING RELIGIOUS DISCUSSION

If waiting produces no real opening for religious dialogue, it then becomes the minister's task to initiate such discussion. This is consistent with the missionary character of New Testament faith. We are to go into the world and preach the gospel to every creature, to make disciples of all nations. None of us--hospital chaplains, pastors, or lay persons--are exempt from this responsibility.

But what of the anxiety we are likely to arouse in patients? Is this not destructive of their total well-being? Should terminally ill patients, who are weakened, vulnerable, and depressed, be disturbed by the intrusion of the religious question? The answers to these questions probably depend on one's concept of anxiety. Most behavioral scientists would agree that excessive anxiety is destructive, but that some anxiety is necessary for change and growth. Oates (1958) writes, "Yet the cross itself presents the most intense anxiety of all, the tension of an impending birth of a new life." Later Oates (1958) quotes the comfort of Thomas à Kempis: "'When thou art ill at ease and troubled is the time when thou are nearest unto blessing.'" Some anxiety is necessary for new birth.

Each initiative should include sensitivity to the patient, and should be made in such a way that it can easily be turned aside. Our authority in the sick room increases in proportion to our acceptance of responsibility. What words should we use? Certainly no hard and fast rule can be laid down. Three arts come to mind as, perhaps, being appropriate: the arts of wondering, of imagining, and of supposing. With Jed White, I wondered aloud if Jed had been thinking of God and how God might be related to him in his illness. He responded that he had been thinking about this a lot.

A MINISTRY OF INTRODUCTION

The Church of England Commission on Evangelism has written, "To evangelize is to so present Christ Jesus in the power of the Holy Spirit, that men shall come to put their trust in God through Him, to accept Him as their Savior, and serve Him as their King in the fellowship of His Church" (Southard 1962).

To a Jed White, how does one "present Christ Jesus in the power of the Holy spirit?" How does one begin a ministry of introduction? With Jed, my approach was heavily dependent on his own tradition. After encouraging Jed to express his own understanding of what it means to become a Christian, I shared my own understanding with Jed. I pointed to Jed's need for confession and repentance toward God and the possibility of his acceptance of Christ as Savior. I used First John (1:9 and 1:12) as supporting Scriptures. I worked hard at answering Jed's questions and clarifying my earlier explanation. Finally, I suggested that Jed think about these matters and told him that I would return later.

THE FREE DECISION

On the whole, modern evangelistic methods seek an immediate decision and "instant salvation": if you have a prospective convert at a revival meeting, get him down the aisle; if you are witnessing face to face, press for an immediate decision. In other words, "Don't let the fish off the hook." Although it is not the purpose of this chapter to analyze or evaluate such methods, I suggest the obvious, that to treat human beings in this manner is not only highly manipulative, but reflects little faith in the real power of the gospel.

In working with Jed White, I wanted him to have time to reflect and to make a free decision. After allowing this time I returned, willing to accept whatever decision he had made. Jed's desire to become a Christian was followed by a prayer of confession and commitment. For Jed, it was necessary to suggest words of prayer.

BAPTISM, CONVERSION, AND CHRISTIAN GROWTH

My own tradition is renowned for "dunking and dropping" its new converts. I was determined that this would not happen to Jed. Following Jed's conversion, I took some responsibility for his growth. There was no indication that Jed's new church, some 60 miles from his home, ever assumed such responsibility. I did fail, however, to provide Jed with an opportunity to partake of the Lord's Supper.

CONCLUSION

Do hospital chaplains and pastors have any responsibility to witness to unchurched, terminally ill patients? The perspective provided here answers this question affirmatively. The guidelines I suggest include an implicit initial approach, pastoral patience, sensitive raising of the religious issue, a ministry of introduction, the allowance of a free decision, and attention to the patient's baptism, communion, and Christian growth.

REFERENCES

Oates, W.E. Anxiety in Christian Experience, p. 118. Philadelphia: Westminster Press, 1955.

---. The Bible in Pastoral Care, p. 19. Philadelphia: Westminster Press, 1958.

Southard, S. Pastoral Evangelism, pp. 7, 8. Nashville: Broadman Press, 1962.

---. Pastoral Evangelism, pp. 60, 72. Atlanta: John Knox Press, 1981.

20

The Memorial Service in a Hospital Setting

David C. Koch

1. The accident was horrible! Seven members of one extended family were killed in their station wagon. The truck driver said that they just pulled right out in front of him. There was nothing he could do. The only survivor was a 12-year-old boy who was admitted to the intensive-care unit of Burlington County Memorial Hospital. Fortunately for the boy, his father was not in the car, but was at work. In spite of his terrible anguish and disbelief, the father could do what was necessary. The boy, with his legs in traction, could do nothing. They were a strong Roman Catholic family. The funeral Mass was poignant. I went on behalf of the boy and recorded the service, including the priest's mention of the names of all those who had died. That helped to confirm the reality for the boy, but what could he do to participate in the expression and accomplishment of his own grief? Could he put it at rest and move on? I encouraged him to go to the cemetery after his release from the hospital, but I wondered if there were something more we could do here in the hospital.

2. The woman was only 36 years old. Her six children were all in school, although the youngest had just begun. Life had been a struggle for them even before the woman and her husband had been divorced. But in a hopeful way, the discovery of her bone cancer had brought them closer together again. At least the father had rallied to the role of care-giver, and the children would be all right. However, no one was talking. The children had only been allowed to come to the hospital to see their mother a couple of times. She didn't want them to see her like that, she said, with the unexpressed hope that she would soon get better. She didn't. She died, and her children had to face that horrible truth.

Both the chaplain and the social worker had worked closely
with the woman, but she wasn't ready to confide in the children until it was too late. The family had long before separated from a religious-support community. What could we do
from within the hospital?

3. She had worked in housekeeping on the same floor
of the hospital to which she was admitted. One of her co-
workers had found her slumping on the floor of a utility clos-
et. It looked like a devastating stroke. She wasn't very old,
but she had been struggling with high blood pressure for
quite a while. She came around at first, regaining at least
enough consciousness to open her eyes and look pleadingly
at her family, who exploded in their own anguish: Couldn't
we do more? She worked here! Shouldn't she get better treatment? If she were a doctor, the nurses would be more attentive! She had been getting better, she might even have gone
home soon, and now she has lost consciousness again. The
nurses did what they could after the second stroke as fully
as they had done after the first. The family knew it, but
couldn't feel it. The chaplain stood with them as she died,
just as he had ministered to them all during her hospitalization. Again I wondered if we could we give them a fuller opportunity to express and work through their anger and loss,
especially since they were part of our hospital family?

The repetition of similar cases innumerable times began
to make a significant impact on my thinking about what and
how much we were doing in our ministry before, during, and
after patients' deaths. Our program included full-time and
part-time clinical pastoral education, an on-call community
clergy program to deal with overnight emergencies, and several lay volunteers who made friendly visitations. What was
clear, however, was that time and time again patients exhibited signs of incomplete or blocked grief that were detrimen-
tal to their wholeness. Patients were hurting because of
previous grief, families were hurting because of current
grief; the staff were hurting for both reasons.

The basic criterion for a successful grief experience is
the movement from attachment to the person who has died
toward reentry into the fullness of life without that person.
The bereaved must turn a corner, leaving behind as a historical experience the life of the person who has died, with
its particular meaning and needs, and stepping toward a new
life that has meaning and needs without that person. The
process may take the form of reintegrating the part of the
self that was transferred or projected onto the person who
died. It may require more wholeness than was present in or
possible for the grieving person before the separation forced
by death. The opportunity for the survivor is growth in
wholeness. The danger is the incorporation into the self of
the disintegration that separation by death symbolizes.

It seemed, therefore, that those of us in the hospital setting, where death in our society is so often focused, could take steps to facilitate the turning of that corner. It seemed, too, from the perspective of pastoral care or theology, that we should take whatever steps we could. The theological foundation of pastoral care can be perceived as being about the first business of life, which is the pilgrimage toward a wholeness that confirms, accepts, and rejoices in each individual whom God has created. As the leader of a pastoral-care department, I had the opportunity to assist the grief process further. With the assistance of a group of full-time, summer, clinical pastoral-education students, the blessing of our chaplaincy advisory committee, and the legal sanction of our hospital's counselor, we proceeded to develop our memorial service program.

The memorial service was to serve several purposes. First, we proposed to provide a corner-turning event. Second, we wanted to give an opportunity for grieving persons to share in the company of others who were experiencing loss, so that the isolation of bereavement could be broken. Third, we wanted to reaffirm the reality of the loss each person had experienced by confirming the name of the one who had died. Fourth, we wanted to give those who grieved an opportunity to give the life of the one who died to their God, and thereby to confirm the significance and acceptance of that life in both its scope and its limits. Finally, we wanted to share in this experience as hospital personnel who had come into intimate contact with those who had died and those who remained. We are part of those who remain after each death. And each death is a grief experience for us, too.

The first memorial service was conducted during August 1980. Those invited were the families of patients who had died in the hospital or in the emergency room during the previous two months. There had been approximately 100 deaths during that time. The hospital staff was also invited to participate. To notify people of this first service, we sent a letter over my signature, and when possible made followup telephone calls. The letter was a form that was personalized by the inside address and salutation and by reference to the relationship of the person who had died to the recipient of the letter. The service was held on a Monday evening and led by the four students and myself. Fifty-one persons attended the first service, far more than we ever imagined would come. Among them were the six children of the two women mentioned above. After the service, light refreshments were served and those attending were given the opportunity to stay and share with each other and the chaplains in further grief work. The majority of those attending stayed.

The response to the first pilot service was very encouraging, and indicated we had attained our goals. Indeed, no negative criticism of the experience was received. Although I was aware that such overwhelming support might hide suppressed feelings, the positive responses have kept coming in. Of special significance to me was the unsolicited letter to the editor of a local paper in which one woman described her experience at the service. Subsequently, another local paper interviewed me and the letter-writer extensively, during which she eloquently expressed the impact of the service. I quote from this latter article:

> The people around Joanne tried to help. . . .
> They assured her that she was young, that
> someday she would marry again, that time
> would heal . . . And you know what? It was
> the last thing I wanted to hear . . . I needed
> people to say "Hey, it's O.K. to grieve--some-
> thing awful has happened to you. Don't run
> from it."

> About a month after Mike's death Joanne got
> a letter from the chaplain's office . . . in-
> viting her to a unique service. At that point
> she was as dazed and agonized as she has
> [sic] ever been . . . and the thought of at-
> tending a memorial service . . . at the hos-
> pital in which he had died seemed repugnant.
> Too difficult. Almost bizarre.

> But Joanne . . . thought . . . and finally
> realized that . . . "if someone wanted to
> honor Mike . . . I wanted to be there." She
> invited members of her family. . . .

> "It was one of the best things that has hap-
> pened to me . . . It gave Mike's death
> meaning and dignity--it gave me a chance to
> see that I wasn't alone, that others were
> suffering too.

> "It was a kind of marker for me, a chance
> to face Mike's death and not hide from it. I
> think I came away from that service finally
> realizing that this had happened, that it was
> real."

The service has successfully met almost all of the goals we intended for it. The one it has not met in its current form is the integration of staff into the sharing, grieving process with families. Very few staff have attended.

Problems with the services have centered on the administrative and organizational areas. It is essential that complete listings of deaths be obtained and that all names be spelled accurately. The letter of invitation seems to work best when an original is sent to each family, but this requires extensive secretarial service or a repeating typewriter. My dependence on volunteers to prepare the letters has necessitated the use of duplicated copies with the appropriate inside address and salutation added to each one. Additional office supply costs are caused by the secretarial time and the paper supplies used. It has seemed best, in our experience, to keep up with deaths weekly but not to send the letters until about three weeks before each service, catching up with the latest deaths just the week before the service.

The worship service itself has been kept simple and as ecumenical as possible. Burlington County Memorial Hospital is in a usual religious setting for the United States, but has a relatively small Jewish population. The central features of the service, other than the overall worship setting, have been the prayer of memorial and the prayer of renewal. During the former, the names of those who died during each week covered by the service are read in alphabetical order and a single candle is lit for each week. During the prayer of renewal, a light from the memorial candles is passed to each of the congregants. We use the kind of candles that are usually passed out at Christmas candlelight services. This transfer of light is intended to symbolize the reintegration of the lives of those who have died in those remaining and the renewal of those lives for living in light rather than darkness.

The memorial service has become an ongoing part of the life of our hospital and a significant ministry of the pastoral-care and education department. Our primary goals of meeting the needs of those in grief more deeply than we did in the past have been met. In addition, the service has provided very positive public relations benefit to the hospital. After each round of invitations to the service, letters are received thanking many in the hospital for their care and continuing concern. The memorial service has been a positive success in the short run. I hope that the long-term benefits for those in bereavement will be as positive.

21

The Angel of Death: Narrative and Its Role in Grief

John L. Topolewski

"Tell me, what happened?" In response to this question or others like it, those of us who grieve begin to create a narrative that gives structure to our experience, articulation to our emotions, and, if carefully crafted, an issue out of our afflictions.

The story we tell becomes, in time, a paradigm of the grief with which we have labored. It is a retrogressive tale that often begins with a review of those events and emotions that surrounded the death, and then begins to reach back into the past, developing some semblance of chronology and attempting to establish some overall perspective on living and dying. It is a story that may take months or years to craft, as we move through the continuum of emotions and understandings that may lead us to various levels of acceptance. Even later, with retelling and refinement, it is a story that may bring a tightness to our throats, a thickening of our speech, and tears to our eyes. Yet, there is grace in such a tale, and such grace comes with the realization that in the pain we can find the cure.

In order to understand how important such a narrative is to our grief, and to understand the positive impact that members of the helping professions--specifically the clergy-- may have on its development, we need to examine why and how such sotries are crafted. To reduce such narratives to their fundamental causality and subsequent structure, we may say that death is the experience, grief is the response, and acceptance or reconciliation is the goal.

Our first task is to deal with the reality of death. The experience can be all too personal and overwhelming. However, it must not be viewed only as an experience that can be factually verified and immediately externalized. Experience involves both encounter and revelation. We are not only confronted with the actuality of death, we are also given some insight into the nature of that actuality and its impact upon us. Understanding might come with the awareness of just how important those who have died have been to us; it might arise from the realization and fear that we too will die; or, to borrow a phrase from the psalmist, understanding may take form in "a heart of wisdom" (Ps. 90:12). Our story is necessitated by death, and it encompasses those revelations we have received.

Experience does not stand alone. It requires a response. To respond to experience is to sort through it or, to use a Kantian phrase, to categorize it in certain specific ways. Experience takes upon itself the first veneer of structure with symbolization. Initially, our response to death may be non-verbal or quasi-verbal, expressed by tears or the ventilation of gross emotion. Soon, however, our response turns to words, the very beginning of our tale. Experience plus symbolization yields meaning. To make some sense of our grief, we begin to craft our story and to manipulate our symbols in ways that may move us into and through our loss. It is precisely at this point, when we are groping for appropriate symbols, struggling to find words that can both describe and give order to our confrontation with death, that those who stand with us in our pain--family, friends, nurses, physicians, and clergy--can be of most help. Our symbolization will be shaped, in part, by the responses of those around us. If only in a secondhand way, every one of us has attempted to find some meaning in death. Although these efforts may be shallow, encapsulated by strong emotions, or even digressive or denying, the meanings of death will be shared. Death demands a response from us all. There is no effective way of screening or blocking the responses of those who stand in its presence.

The potential for care that clergy bring to that time when grief is most intense is contained within the fact that symbols are the stock and trade of a clergyperson's calling. Practice of profession is founded upon symbolization; in the presence of the clergyperson, a presence that is symbolic in itself, we are put in contact with a heritage and tradition rich with metaphors that are both accepting of death and affirming of life. Bondage and liberation, death and resurrection, are the very stories on which our Judeo-Christian heritage has been built. In a variety of ways, these metaphors, as well as others like them or derived from them, can provide helpful ingredients for us as we craft our tale. Members of the clergy, by sharing their stories and their response to death, and by the skillful use of faith's many symbols, can give both help and caring.

A word of caution needs to be introduced at this point, and I speak now from my own experience as a clergyperson who can often be found in the role and position mentioned above. Because of the very nature of stories themselves, when one crafts or tells a story, the hearers are willing, within certain limits, to suspend their critical judgment. Our basic response to a story is one of acceptance and absorption, not criticism and unbelief. Clergy need to remember this, for too often we tend to attempt to demythologize the symbols of these stories and rationalize their content. It is not possible to assume singular meanings for complex metaphors, even when such meanings are ours, or when we assume that these meanings are, or should be, those of the storyteller. Hear these stories in their entirety and, if the choice of symbols is unwise, then retell the tale with appropriate substitutions. Just as we respond to the stories of others, so when we become myth-makers others will respond to us, appropriating what rings true and can be incorporated within their own narrative.

One more word needs to be said about the role clergy play as they seek to enable those of us who grieve to ventilate our emotions and articulate our responses. Narrative can help us to understand where we are in our grief, and can also point us to where we might be. Symbols are pedagogical; stories are experiential, filled with encounter and revelation. I am not suggesting that clergy should artificially superimpose levels of acceptance or reconciliation on those who grieve, but rather that they should hold out acceptance and reconciliation as offerings of grace-bearing metaphors toward which we may move. Stories can model the entire grief process, from denial to acceptance, and such modeling, in times of personal sharing or in funeral homilies, can become expressions of healing, care, and reconciling love.

One such story has undergone many changes in both its oral and written form, yet it continues to speak to and for me. My mother was a tough bird. She lived alone in a small apartment in Jersey City, commuted each day by bus to her job at the bank, and asserted her independence from her two inquisitive sons by insisting that she was "all right." In spite of such protestations, she lived within the confines of a decaying inner city, had her purse snatched, and sensed that special anxiety which comes with the end of daylight. She smoked too much, ate poorly, and saw doctors infrequently.

She was generous to a fault, often setting aside her own needs so that she might do something special for her family. During the preholiday season, she would take a second job in a children's store, and received her pay in clothing that she set aside for her grandchildren. Years ago, before she had faced the unique responsibilities of being what

we now call a single parent, she gave leadership in Parents'
Council, the church, and ward politics. In many ways, she
was a formidable personality, both compelling and worthy of
emulation.

Some time ago, when my brother lived in Nebraska and
I in Pennsylvania, my mother heard a knock at her door.
I'm not sure of the exact time of his arrival, but I do know
that when my mother released the dead-bolt and opened the
door as far as the safety chain permitted, she was able to
see who it was. There he stood, with his yellowed and distorted face: a violator, a rapist, whose name was Cancer.

Mom called, and my brother and I ran to help. We told
her we were strong enough to lean against the door, determined enough to keep back the intruder, able enough to protect and defend her. We laughed; we reminisced; we made
light of her problem, knowing that our mother had resolved
other difficulties so well. But when she was not looking we
parted the curtains, pulled back the edge of the shade, and
saw him standing, still waiting, on the stoop.

Time passed, and the demands of family and employment
drew both my brother and me back to our homes and jobs.
In some ways, it was a relief. Doing something took some of
the edge from our anger and fear. Somehow we tried to lose
ourselves within the parochial concerns of everyday life,
hoping against hope that there might be some reversal of our
future. And then the phone rang again.

My mother had responded to another knock at her door.
This time she was slower to answer, frightened by her first
encounter, but she had no real choice except to look through
the little crack that the safety chain afforded. There he
stood again, with his grim and distorted countenance, with
his withered and discolored hands, with a presence both awesome and strangely patient. And his name--his name was
Terminal.

Again we came to lean against the door. We were not
as sure of ourselves as before, but we did not let on either
to each other or to Mom. We tried to be sons even when our
mother became our daughter. We tried to be realistic even
when our planning was aborted by our guilt. And when she
was not looking, we parted the curtains, pulled back the
edge of the shade, and discovered that he was still there.

Then, in the very early hours of the morning when we
were to celebrate the birthday of my oldest daughter (Mom's
first grandchild), we heard the knock again. We ran to the
door, willing to lean against it with all our might, straining
to defend, her only protection against the intruder. But in
the very moment that we rushed toward the door, we heard
our mother's voice, strangely firm, reminiscent of an old
authority, calm and resolved. "Step aside," she said. "Open
the door and let him in." We could no longer resist and, in
spite of our worst fears, we opened the door.

There he stood. And he was changed. The ugly visage of the Angel of Death had been transformed into something, someone oddly attractive, even beautiful. He came to our mother and held out his hands. He offered two gifts, Peace and Rest. And then, on a day now remembered for both birthing and dying, our mother went with the Angel.

Then shall come to pass the saying that is written: "Death is swallowed up in victory." "O Death, where is they victory? O Death, where is thy sting?" [I Corinthians 15:54-55]

22

Pastoral-Care Issues in Experiences of Loss, Death, and Bereavement

Samuel Lucius Gandy

The occurrence of death, the event of a family loss, and the woe of grief are human factors, and as such are common in mankind. This chapter is limited to U.S. society, and more particularly the black population. The primary question is whether loss, death, and bereavement find a unique expression and adjustment among blacks. Is there something within their cultural context that cushions the shocks of loss and of death in greater degree than in the larger population? Is there such a thing as acclimated suffering in which the element of endurance eases the pain?

Human bondage so completely restricts the movements of persons and groups that only the human imagination can rescue individuals from pits of despair and caverns of alienation. It has been quite well established that the sensitive imagination of Afro-American slaves, woven into their religious faith, rescued them from inner emptiness and social isolation. They sang themselves into fresh and vigorous meanings for being (Frankl 1959) and projected themselves by their imagination into worlds of assurance and newness of being. Compensatory elements in religious faith provided the guarantees that life can transcend the existential circumstances of raw denial of worth (Mays 1938).

Antebellum preachers, though untutored, intuitively afforded the primary focus in pastoral care--the significance of the individual and the necessary establishment of personal worth. As difficult as this requirement was in a closed human system, it was, nevertheless, achieved. The resulting social character in the slave communities was one in which sufferings were not absolute disintegrators of character: sufferings could be endured and surmounted; the shocks in human existence were not final; and the everyday occurrence of death and other losses to family or community were interpreted

against a background of vital religious faith. Since slave society was essentially classless, the element of suffering became a factor in social character, making endurance central.
It is still a continuing quality of survival among the Afro-
American masses.

Of course, human suffering is human suffering, and
the slaves were not unique in their interpretation and expression of this element of the human condition. In fact, it is
reasonable to assume that the Hebrew cultural experience as
stated in the Old Testament was a source of inspiration for
the antebellum Afro-American slave: "Didn't My Lord Deliver
Daniel?"

It is to be assumed that human suffering interpreted
in a pattern of religious beliefs affords a dimension for encountering the tragic that may not be found in any other
way. Since slavery or legal segregation and customary social
discrimination create classless and uniform social living conditions, a social character may emerge that seems characteris-
tic in the depth of its social expression. Conversely, as
bondage lessens or loses control, the depth of sensitivity to
the tragic may also lessen or evaporate. This response may
be seen in the contemporary class status system, in which
social mobility has been enhanced by socioeconomic gains for
the individual.

There is significant carryover of the essence of this
element among the congregations of black churches, indicat-
ing that a distinction can be drawn between minority congregations and more privileged congregations in their capacity
to absorb grief and loss. It is the constancy of the tragic
and the intensity of need that makes long-suffering a more
disciplined factor among the disinherited and underprivileged.
Ghettos, on the whole, know no thin lines of privacy and
privilege. Every situation or condition seems to be of immediate neighborly concern. The caring process is a constant universal concern in ghettos; pastors and people are present to
each other. Antebellum and postbellum black preachers arti-
culated the compensatory role of religion. Therefore, the
dread of death was not always a threatening presence, and
life after death was seen as a joyful state of being. Pastoral
care was highlighted in funeral sermons in which the good
and the beautiful erased the evil and the ugly. There was a
literal wrapping of oneself around the bereaved family with
strongly felt responses. Loss was never experienced alone;
neighborly assurances were always present, before and after
death. They were made concrete by the giving and sharing
of food, clothing, housing, money, and whatever else seemed
to be needed. Such sharing is not likely where social distance prevails and where token expression of support is so-
ciably accepted. Genuine presence means all of the way.

The funeral itself is a different kind of institution among the disinherited masses. It is not simply that there is burial, but the way it is done. The compensatory factor finds an outlet here also. There is a kind of exhibitionism that takes place. Poverty is momentarily supplanted in order to provide a truly decent "going away" for the dead. Here again, pastoral care is personal, direct, and graphically reassuring. The plantation pastor-preacher and the big-city church leader have much in common in times of loss, death, and bereavement--the funeral occasion and the compensatory. This kind of deep personal involvement may not find practice in the middle and upper classes.

The managing of grief is an individual requirement, but the sharing of grief by pastor and congregation makes the individual responsibility manageable. Shared grief before and after the funeral is not a casual social task among church populations of the masses but a moral requirement that is taken seriously. It is a neighborly task that springs from the roots of religious faith. It is regrettable that instruments for measuring the degree of such sharing among the less privileged are not included herein. The approach is one of observation and of historical continuity recorded in the history of a people.

REFERENCES

Frankl, V.E. Man's Search for Meaning. New York: Washington Square Press, 1959.

Mays, B.E. The Negro's God. Boston: Chapman and Grimes, 1938.

23

Loss, Grief, and Anticipation of Death in the Elderly

J. P. Pollard

In 1974, in response to an increasing number of requests from church groups and ministers about their involvement with elderly nursing-home patients, a pastoral counselor
and I set about learning the needs of these patients by listening to the patients themselves. The rising interest in
thanatology had led a number of local clergy to search for
ways to minister most effectively to this group. They began,
as we did, with the assumption that such patients were
heavily involved in anticipatory grief.

With the cooperation of the director of a local nursing
home, we were able to schedule a weekly group for residents.
These numbered 145 men and women, predominately elderly
and ambulatory. The residents were informed by the management that a weekly "talk group" would meet in the cafeteria
and that those who wished to attend would be assisted in
reaching the cafeteria. Each weekly session lasted approximately 1.5 hours. We began each session with Kool-Aid and
cookies in an effort to create a comfortable, nonthreatening
atmosphere. The number of patients who attended meetings
ranged between 12 and 26, with the average about 20.

A feeling of closeness soon developed among those in
the group. When situational crises arose, such as the serious
illness or death of a resident, the focus of the group spon-
taneously fixed on the crisis. Conversations would grow out
of group members' thoughts and feelings about the affected
individual. This typically led into a discussion of their own
feelings.

As group leaders, we took the stance of hosts, friends,
and facilitators. We came with no fixed agenda and no objective other than to encourage group participants to talk
about the things that concerned them. We occasionally inter-
vened if a member of the group attempted to monopolize the

session. It was usually sufficient to open a session with a
question, such as "What do you think about when you are in
a nursing home?" or "Has anything happened this week you
would like to talk about?" We did no therapy or didactic work
with the group. We felt they would benefit from their mutual
sharing and that we could best learn from them in a casual
setting.

It soon became apparent that we were incorrect in our
premise that these people were struggling with anticipatory
grief. We observed symptoms of grief, such as guilt, depression, tears, and anger, but these seemed to be reactions to
losses other than those associated with impending death. We
were able to summarize the losses that group members had
experienced. These losses could be placed in three catego-
ries: (1) loss of symbols and familiar locale, (2) loss of power, and (3) loss of meaning.

We observed the loss of symbols in a variety of ways.
For most, the loss of the "home place" was significant. We
were repeatedly reminded how much people's homes become a
part of their self-images. This loss had brought a variety of
associated losses, such as the loss of ability to play host to
family gatherings, to prepare favorite foods, and to have
pets and other symbols of personal definition. The group
verbalized feelings not unlike those of the ancient Jews, of
whom the biblical writer declared, "They hung up their
harps upon the willows and wept, saying 'How can we sing
the songs of Zion in a strange land?'" However warm, bright,
and cheerful the nursing home was made to be, it remained a
"strange land" to most of those in the group.

Loss of power was also apparent. Our society places
great emphasis on power as a determinant of personal worth.
Consciously and unconsciously, success tends to be equated
with one's ability to control people and processes. One elderly man declared to the group, "I used to be a road boss for
the county, those guys had to jump when I told them to."
The tone of his voice indicated that whatever power he once
possessed was now gone, and that he felt a sense of power-
lessness. Those who used to control their schedules and
destinies now found themselves conforming to the controls of
the management of the nursing home. The normal degree of
regimentation typically present in institutional living was
frequently a target for the residents' resentment and hostility. We observed that loss of power and control was a very
real source of grief for the members of the group.

Another highly significant loss for the group members
was the loss of meaning in their lives. The Protestant work
ethic declares that "idle hands are the devil's workshop."
Those who follow this philosophy as long as they are young
can avoid housing the devil by staying busy. But when people are old and confined to nursing homes, idleness becomes

a fact of life. We encountered grief in many residents that
seemed directly related to their loss of a sense of meaning in
their lives. At various times, we heard residents lament
their inability to do "an honest day's work." Another frequent statement had to do with their puzzlement about why
God had left them on earth, inasmuch as there was no longer
any way for them to be productive. Most group members
identified meaning in life as being able to perform some task.

So it was that after several months with the group, we
concluded that the anger, guilt, depression, and tears we
had observed did not relate to anticipatory grief in the face
of impending death, but rather to these kinds of loss. We
came to understand that there was little fear of death within
the group. Members of the group spoke of death casually,
easily, and at times as though it was a friendly deliverer.
When we deliberately turned conversations toward the subject of death, we found far less tension than in a group of
younger adults. The residents treated death with a casual-
ness that seemed to grow out of their perception of it as a
natural part of life. This was especially true of those who
had lived satisfying lives.

Although we did not observe callousness on the part of
the nursing-home personnel, we thought that most of them
did not understand the residents' expressions of grief for
what they were. Too often, personnel reacted to the symptoms of grief instead of dealing with the sense of loss that
produced those symptoms. In our opinion, a thorough ground-
ing in the dynamics of grief would have been appropriate for
all the employees.

We observed that clergy who were attempting to minister to the residents did so in a rather stereotyped fashion.
The emphasis was usually on the presentation of sermons and
music, to which residents could only listen passively. We
suggested that the clergy consider ways of involving them in
a ministry within the nursing home, for which the residents
themselves would be at least partly responsible. We felt that
more emphasis on religion as action within the sphere of the
living situation was in order. We stressed the importance of
forming a community of mutual care and concern within the
nursing home. It seemed vitally important that the residents'
sense of responsibility be enhanced.

It is very difficult to institutionalize people without de-
priving them of their symbols, power, and meaning in life.
It is even more difficult for people to cope with these losses
without experiencing grief. Perhaps pastoral care should
focus on two goals in a nursing-home setting. First, there
must be an awareness of the undeniable fact that institution-
alization produces grief. This grief must be facilitated and
worked through with residents until they achieve some degree of acceptance. Second, emphasis should be placed on

minimizing these losses whenever and wherever possible. By encouraging residents to personalize their rooms with familiar objects, to make their own choice of dress, and to engage in social life, the loss of symbols could be made less devastating. A considerable amount of creative work could be done in this area. If residents were encouraged to become involved in the affairs of the nursing home, and perhaps in some kind of self-government and regulation, they could maintain a sense of power in some aspects of their lives. Effective ministry within the nursing home could also encourage the formation of a sort of community concern with attendant responsibilities and a sense of mission. This would also enhance the residents' sense of meaning and purpose.

As the number of institutionalized older citizens increases, the challenge to those involved in pastoral care also increases. It is a challenge that deserves our best efforts.

24

Grief: The Road to Recovery

Arnaldo Pangrazzi

"My husband was never sick a day in his life. Then, in the turn of five months, he was gone. Since he died, I've spent my nights crying for him. But my tears won't bring him back. I am just lost in the world without him." The woman was crying. Someone in the group put an arm around her shoulder and gave her a handkerchief.

"I know how you feel," commented a voice from another corner of the room. "It gets so lonely at times, you want to die, too. I find myself asking, 'What is the purpose of life, day after day?' It seems I just go through the motions of waking up, dressing, going to work, coming home . . . but there's no life or meaning to it."

"The hardest part for me," said a young mother, "was the lack of having someone around telling me, 'You are worth something!' All I really need is just to have someone to talk with . . . to remember. My friends seem to avoid bringing up my husband's name. Maybe they are afraid I will break down or start to cry. What do they expect me to do . . . forget him?"

The sharing was intermingled with silence, tears, and laughter. "I'd like to know if other people who have young children are being asked the type of questions my four-year-old son asked me the other day," said a young man. "Whenever a woman comes to the house, he thinks she's going to stay. Yesterday he said, 'Dad, I need a new mom because I want brothers and sisters.' I told him, 'Randy, you've got grandma.' He replied, 'She's not enough.' I sobbed, 'I'll get you a new mom when I find someone like your mother.' I guess he thought I would buy a new mom at the store for a dime." There was a mixture of sadness and affection in the laughter that followed.

These comments came from people participating in a support group for the bereaved, which meets bimonthly under the sponsorship of St. Joseph's Hospital in Milwaukee. The purpose of the group is to create an environment where people who have been hurt by the loss of a loved one can come together to share and support each other. There is a sense of kinship and credibility that people feel for each other when they hurt together.

The death of a loved one is often a major disruption that requires adjustment in our way of looking at the world and our plans for living in it. The reaction to this loss at the physical, emotional, spiritual, and social levels varies from person to person, and depends on the circumstances surrounding the death--the type of relationship that existed between the deceased and the bereaved, the strengths one has, and the quality of one's support system. Certainly a person who can count on a positive self-image, an ability to relate easily, a faith to lean on, and the willingness to take initiative will do much better than a person who has an unclear self-identity, tends to withdraw rather than to engage, has difficulty learning from pain, and is afraid to take risks.

It has been suggested that the pain of grief is the price we have to pay for love. In a very real way, whenever we choose to love someone we are also choosing to be hurt. The time comes when we have to say good-bye, to let go. That is when grief begins.

As it takes time to love, so it also takes time to let go. People say, "Time heals." But time by itself does not heal. If a grieving person sits in a corner waiting for time to take care of bitter sorrow, time won't do anything. It is what we do with time that can heal. The purpose of this chapter is to offer some practical suggestions about what to do with time so that it may become a source of healing.

The biblical image of the exodus can offer us a good point of reference for understanding our grief. The Israelites, like us, experienced the grief of letting go. They had to let go of a place that was familiar. They were confronted with the uncertainty of the future, with the adjustment to a new life-style, with the experience of the desert. They wandered in the desert for 30 years, complaining, struggling, hurting, and hoping. During their desert experience, God gave them the Ten Commandments to guide them in their journey toward the future.

Bereaved people have a taste of that desert experience in their own lives. There is a danger of being stuck in the desert, in their grief. I offer ten commandments, guidelines that can help the bereaved who take time to practice them to find their way to hope, freedom, and healing.

1. Take Time to Accept Death

"My turning point was when I realized and accepted that my husband wasn't going to be there to open my door, and I wasn't going to find him in bed." Acceptance of death remains a condition for living. The pain will never get better until we face it. Often it is hard to realize that what happened has really happened, that life has changed.

Fantasy acts as an anesthetic to soften the pain. We hope it was all a bad dream, that we are going to wake up in the morning and everything will be all right. We hope that our loved one will call us from work, or that we will hear that cherished voice when we step into the house. As the reality of death gradually sinks in, we ask why it happened. It's really not important that we find an answer to that question because the answer is rational and our hurt is emotional. What's important is to realize that it did happen. The only way to deal with death is to accept it. We cannot fight death; we can only embrace it, no matter how painful that might be. Death confronts us with our mortality and vulnerability. We have a firsthand experience of what it means to be helpless, naked, lonely, and hurt . . . of what it means to be truly human. Yes, our loved one has died. But that doesn't mean we have to die too. We have to pick up the pieces and go on from there.

2. Take Time to Let Go

One of the most difficult human experiences is letting go and yet, from birth to death, life is a series of such actions, some temporary, some permanent. Letting go reminds us that we are not in control of life, and that we need to accept what we cannot control. So often we try to play God because it can be so painful to be human, especially in the face of death.

Letting go means adjusting to a new reality in which the deceased is no longer present. And yet, many bereaved people live in an atmosphere that means their loved one has not really died, that life has not really changed. Everything in the house is left as it used to be. They seem to live for the deceased, not for themselves.

Letting go takes place when the "we" becomes "I," when we are able to substitute the physical presence of the deceased with the memories they have left us, when we are able to change the patterns in our lives and in our environments. I remember a widow who used to wake up at night in the gesture of reaching out to her husband, only to discover that he wasn't there. That filled her with grief and kept her awake. She was able to make a significant change by deciding to sleep on his side of the bed. Physical change facilitated her psychological adjustment.

Letting go occurs when we are able to endure and accept the anger, guilt, fear, sadness, depression, or whatever feelings accompany the death. Letting go occurs when we are able to tolerate our helplessness and insecurity, when we are willing to face our fears, to wait, to trust, and to hope again. St. Paul assures us that "We are afflicted, but not crushed; perplexed, but not driven to despair" (1 Cor. 4:8-10).

3. Take Time to Make Decisions

"I am angry at myself for allowing myself to be spoiled. I never took care of the checking account. I never had to make decisions. He did all those things. Now I don't know what to do . . . I feel so helpless." The sense of dependency is echoed in the words of a man who said, "Whenever we went out with friends, my wife used to do all the talking. I just sat back and listened. It's so hard now. People look at me and I just don't know what to say or what topic of conversation to get into." People who have been very dependent on the deceased find themselves lost in the world. They are afraid to give themselves direction, afraid of making mistakes, afraid to ask, afraid to try.

Making mistakes is the way we learn and develop trust in ourselves, especially in unfamiliar areas. It's important that the bereaved be patient with themselves, and gradually learn to make decisions as a way of sustaining their sense of self-worth. It is wise to postpone major decisions. Small decisions are the most important ones to make, from writing out a schedule for the day to setting up tasks to be done.

Planning the day has to do with looking forward to something, whether it is the visit of a friend or a vacation. Looking forward balances that attitude of "I don't want to do anything," or "There is nothing that makes me happy" that often depresses and paralyzes people. Making decisions about our lives helps us gain some control over them and increases our self-confidence.

4. Take Time to Share

"No one, friends or family, cares to remember or cry with us anymore. It's like you want to shout it out to the ceiling: 'Talk to me, talk to me!'" The speaker was one of 25 parents who had gathered together to remember their children and share their grief. When we lose a child, we grieve over the loss of our future. When we lose a spouse, we grieve over the loss of our present. When we lose a parent, we grieve over the loss of our past. The greatest need of those who are bereaved is to have someone to share their pain, memories, and sadness. In life, we can only accept what we can share. Bereaved people need others who will give them time and space to grieve. At times, the comments of well-meaning friends can be insensitive and hurtful:

> "Come on, it has been six months. You should
> be over it by now."

> "He's gone; forget it!"

> "The past is a closed book now."

When we are strangers to grief, it is easy to place our expectations on the bereaved when it becomes too uncomfortable for us to walk with them at their pace. I like the words of a widower who learned to make his wishes known to his friends: "I like to talk about Dorothy. I miss her touch, her presence. But talking about her helps me. I makes me happy to remember her."

Our children are not necessarily the people with whom to share grief. Children tend to look forward, not backward. Particularly during the early stages of grieving, we might need someone who looks backward, because the past, not the future, remains the greatest source of comfort at that time. Trusted friends can be the people who accept us as we are and to whom we can open our hearts.

Sharing memories and feelings with people who are grieving themselves is especially helpful and therapeutic. We learn to understand that our experience is normal, we become aware of different ways of coping, and we realize that the answers to our pain and our lives lie within us as we become free to give and receive in an open, caring way.

5. Take Time to Believe

To survive is to find meaning in suffering. Suffering that has meaning is endurable. However, meaning does not just happen. It takes time, openness, and faith to find positive and redeeming values in our suffering. It's important to realize that God is in the midst of our suffering. "We know that in everything God works for good with those who love Him" (Rom. 8:28).

It is also important to discover the ministry of suffering as a binding power with others who suffer. That's when suffering gives birth to new opportunity through the spirituality of wounded healers. This spirituality is well expressed in a prayer used in the memorial services offered periodically at St. Joseph's Hospital in Milwaukee:

> Our sorrow reminds us that life is not meant
> to avoid pain and that to love is to accept the
> risk of hurting. Help us, O Lord, to gain
> wisdom through our sufferings and give us
> patience and time to work through our feelings.

Help us trust your presence in the events we
do not understand. Put us in touch with the
inner resources hidden in us and guide us
through the future by gently transforming our
grief into compassion, our hurts into new hope
for others.

At times, our grief can shake our faith. We wonder
what God is up to, whether He has forgotten us. We may
even be angry at Him for what we perceive that He has done
to us. Often it becomes difficult to go to church, to pray,
to go on living. The only way out of the desert is to go
through it, trusting that God is there with us. For many
people, religion, with its rituals, the promise of an afterlife,
and its community of support, offers a comforting and
strengthening base in the lonely encounter with helplessness and hopelessness. Our faith does not take away our
grief, but it helps us live with it.

6. Take Time to Forgive

The feeling of guilt and the need for forgiveness accompany many of our experiences, especially those that remain unfinished. We feel guilty about what we did or didn't
do, the clues we missed, the things we said or failed to say.
In reviewing one's life and one's relationship with the deceased, there will always be things that seem to have been
less than ideal. We need to accept our imperfections and
make peace with ourselves. We cannot judge our yesterday
with the knowledge of today. Torturing ourselves for things
we did and wish we hadn't done, or dwelling on the things
we didn't do doesn't change anything. It only makes us miserable.

We need to put our lives into perspective and accept
what has been. Our love for the deceased wasn't perfect; it
included our weaknesses as well as our strengths, and those
of the deceased. Our loved ones have not become holy because they have died. We don't need to idealize them. It's
healthy to remember them as they were.

The need for forgiveness emerges when we are angry.
Here are the words of one mother: "I feel like I have a big
sign on me: 'My son committed suicide.' I am angry at him
and will never forgive him for what he did to our family."

We might be angry at our in-laws because they disap-
peared after the funeral. We might be angry at people because of their comments, insensitivity, or avoidance of us.
We certainly need to own and express our anger. However,
there must also be a time for forgiveness, or the anger can
become destructive and alienating. The last thing that Jesus
did on the cross was to forgive His enemies, "for they do
not know what they are doing." We need to find strength,

through time, to forgive ourselves and others, to forgive life
for hurting us, to forgive death for taking our loved one.

7. Take Time to Feel Good about Yourself

Bereaved people are not sentenced to unhappiness. We
are not born happy or unhappy. We learn to be happy by
the ways we adjust to life crises and use the opportunities
life gives us.

At first, grief confronts us with a number of unpleasant discoveries. All of a sudden, many things seem to go
wrong, from the refrigerator that doesn't work to the faucet
that leaks, from the meal that doesn't taste right to the laun-
dry that doesn't look clean. We need to be patient and to
give ourselves time to learn, time to make mistakes. Especially, we need to affirm ourselves, patting ourselves on the
back for every small thing we learn to do, whether it is re-
placing a light bulb or installing the storm windows. Every
time we do something new, we expand ourselves. We grow
beyond where we were and develop more confidence in the
person we are becoming. I remember the excitement of a
young widow who said: "I went to the library and borrowed
this book on how to do things around the house. I decided
to wallpaper my kitchen. You should see it! It really turned
out pretty good. I was so proud of myself."

The death of a loved one affects our life-style and
changes our self-image. Grief can rapidly shape us and help
us discover a new independence and outlook. This is reflected in the words of a mother: "I am no longer the person I
used to be. I've changed. I believe that my child now has a
better mother because I am more tolerant and accepting. Before, everything had to be just right."

The process of building self-confidence is often sustained by being able to hold a job or keeping busy. It is
also enhanced by other equally important factors, such as
exploring new interests (reading, writing, or taking academic
courses), developing new hobbies (swimming, dancing, yoga,
or gardening), and taking advantage of new opportunities
(traveling or doing volunteer work). All these activities can
help the bereaved reinvest their energies in new endeavors
that provide a feeling of newness, satisfaction, and pleasure.

8. Take Time to Meet New Friends

"I had 570 people at the funeral home. They all offered
to help. Where are they now, six months down the pike?"
The comment of this person reflects the feelings of many bereaved people who feel let down or uncared for by their
friends. The loneliness that is present in grief may be nature's way of mending our broken hearts. Loneliness can also
be transformed into solitude. That happens when we are not

oppressed by our loneliness, but learn to live creatively with it by expanding our self-understanding and inner resources.

We need to reach out. We cannot avoid social contacts because of the imperfections of those we meet. We cannot devalue all relationships except the one that has been lost. Healing occurs when those who are grieving make the first step out of their safe boundaries and invest in others. Old friends may offer security and comfort; new friends will offer opportunities. We can meet new friends through support groups, card clubs, classes, and other activities. A widower who had just attended a support group for the bereaved expressed his feelings: "This group did wonders for me. At first, I was apprehensive. I felt I was entering a room full of strangers. I left with the feeling I was in a room full of friends. Some of these people have become my best friends."

Widows and widowers often feel that they have lost their sense of belonging, that they no longer fit into our couple-oriented society. Thus, they need to find a new sense of belonging. Dating remains helpful in the recovery process because it reminds the bereaved they are liked and appreciated. However, it might be dangerous to try to stop the pain or the hurting by compulsive involvements or remarriage. On the road to recovery, we need friends, not partners. The best way to find a friend is to be one. Like a smile, it returns to you.

9. Take Time to Laugh

"I used to resent people who were happy and laughed. I wanted to scream, 'Why do you laugh? Don't you know I am here? Don't you know what happened?' I felt that way until a friend of mine told me, 'Remember you were laughing, too, when someone else around might have felt miserable.'" In life there are as many reasons to laugh as there are to cry. In grief, a time comes when our tears come with less frequency and intensity, and we learn to remember without crying. Laughter, on the other hand, helps us survive and to reenter life. For someone who has been sad and depressed, there is no better medicine than the ability to smile again. We can smile at memories that come to us. We can laugh at mistakes we've made, things we have said, thoughts we have entertained. There is a lot of comedy in our tragedies. Without laughter and humor, life would indeed become a sad journey.

Laughter is truly one of God's greatest blessings. It helps us accept our limitations, and it develops hope in the present. Laughter defines our movement from helplessness to hopelessness. It is somewhat reflected in the contrasting attitudes of one who wakes up saying, "Oh, God, it's morning" and another who is optimistic and says, "Good morning, God."

Laughter frees us from tension and helps us conserve energy. It takes only 14 muscles to smile and 72 to frown. So it's important that we give ourselves the benefit of relaxing and laughing when we can without feeling guilty. Indeed, when we find ourselves laughing, we are on our way to healing. Then there is hope for us.

10. Take Time to Give

The best way to overcome loneliness and pain is to be concerned about the loneliness and pain of others. People turn away from grief when they feel wanted and needed by the living. Being able to help someone gives us meaning, makes us feel good. It makes us realize that our experience can be placed at the service of others. If you find someone who needs you, that will be your opportunity for healing. Here's how one person phrased it: "This time of grief in my life has probably been the time when I've given more of myself than at any other time. I don't think I'll be able to give as much again."

Being involved with others gives us the feeling that life goes on, and it takes us away from self-pity. Listening to someone, empathizing and sharing over the telephone, providing information, going out for lunch together, are all ways to give of ourselves. We accumulate tremendous wisdom through our encounters with grief, and it needs to be shared.

Healing takes place when we turn our pain into a positive experience, and when we realize that helping others is the key to helping ourselves. When that happens, our problems don't look so big. We expand our newly found strengths and discover that although one door has closed, many others have opened. Recovery from grief requires that we take time to do those things that will enable us to give a renewed meaning to our lives. That's when our journey through grief becomes a journey of discovering ourselves, our potentials, and our resources in the encounter with life. That's when we become better people rather than bitter people. In grief, no one can take away our pain because no one can take away our love. The call of life is to learn to love again.

Index

About the Editors and Contributors

Editors

REV. BRIAN P. O'CONNOR, M.Div., M.P.H., Pastor, Blessed Sacrament Church, Bronx, New York

DR. DANIEL J. CHERICO, Assistant Professor, Department of Health Care and Public Health, C. W. Post Center, Long Island University, Greenvale, New York

CHAPLAIN CAROLE E. SMITH TORRES, Pastoral Associate, Department of Pastoral Care, The Presbyterian Hospital in the City of New York; Conservative Baptist Mission Society, Staten Island, New York

DR. AUSTIN H. KUTSCHER, President, The Foundation of Thanatology; Professor of Dentistry (in Psychiatry), Department of Psychiatry, College of Physicians and Surgeons, Columbia University; Professor of Dentistry (in Psychiatry), School of Dental and Oral Surgeons, Columbia University, New York, New York

RABBI JACOB GOLDBERG, Director, Pastoral Commission on Bereavement and Counseling, New York, New York

DR. KARIN M. MURASZKO, Senior Resident in Neurosurgery, Columbia Presbyterian Medical Center, New York, New York

Contributors

REV. PERRY H. BIDDLE, D. Min., Pastor, First Presbyterian Church, Old Hickory, Tennessee

LEWIS PENHALL BIRD, PH.D., Eastern Regional Director, Christian Medical Society, Haverton, Pennsylvania

CHAPLAIN JOSEPH P. DULANY (LTC), Department of Ministry and Pastoral Care, Walter Reed Army Medical Center, Washington, D.C.

DR. SAMUEL LUCIUS GANDY, Howard University Divinity School, Washington, D.C.

AUDREY K. GORDON, M.A., Psychologist; Lecturer in Psychiatry, Loyola University Stritch School of Medicine, Chicago, Illinois; Member, Board of Directors, Chicago

Area Jewish Hospice Association; Counselor in Death Education, Evanston, Illinois

REV. GARY L. HARBAUGH, Ph.D., Trinity Lutheran Seminary, Columbus, Ohio

REV. WILBUR H. HUGUEY, Clinical Chaplaincy Department, Iowa Methodist Medical Center, Des Moines, Iowa

REV. GORDON E. JACKSON, Professor of Pastoral Care, Pittsburgh, Theological Seminary, Pittsburgh, Pennsylvania

REV. DAVID C. KOCH, Burlington County Memorial Hospital, Mt. Holly, New Jersey

LILLIAN G. KUTSCHER, Publications Editor, The Foundation of Thanatology, New York, New York

REV. EDWARD J. MAHNKE, M.Div., D.D., Director, Chaplaincy and Pastoral Education, The University of Texas M.D. Anderson Hospital and Tumor Institute, Houston, Texas

REV. WILLIAM C. MAYS, D.Min., Chief, Chaplaincy Service, Veterans Administration Medical Center, Nashville, Tennessee; Assistant Professor of Pastoral Theology and Counseling, Vanderbilt Divinity School, Nashville, Tennessee

REV. THOMAS McGOWAN, Ph.D., Associate Professor of Religious Studies, Manhattan College, Riverdale, New York

RABBI STEVEN A. MOSS, Spiritual Leader, B'nai Israel Reform Temple, Oakdale, New York; Coordinator of Jewish Chaplaincy Services, Memorial Sloan-Kettering Cancer Center, New York, New York

FATHER ARNALDO PANGRAZZI, Chaplain, St. Joseph's Hospital, Milwaukee, Wisconsin

CHAPLAIN J. P. POLLARD, Sparks Regional Medical Center, Fort Smith, Arkansas

REV. EDMOND ROBILLARD, O.P., Faculty of Theology, University of Montreal, Montreal, Quebec, Canada

REV. VIRGINIA A. SAMUEL, Assistant Dean, Drew Theological School, Madison, New Jersey

REV. WILLIAM B. SMITH, S.T.D., Professor of Moral Theology and Dean, St. Joseph's Seminary, Yonkers, New York

REV. ROBERT H. SPRINGER, S.J., New York, New York

REV. JOHN L. TOPOLEWSKI, Pastor, Christ United Methodist Church, Mountaintop, Pennsylvania

REV. JEFFREY A. WATSON, Th.M., Ph.D., Washington Bible College, Lanham, Maryland

D. T. WESSELLS, JR., Ed.D., Counseling Supervisor, Associates in Lynnhaven, Virginia Beach, Virginia

REV. HAROLD D. YARRINGTON, Chief Chaplain/Director of Clinical Pastoral Education, Connecticut Valley Hospital, Middletown, Connecticut